Understanding
Experimental
Pharmacology

Understanding
Experimental
Pharmacology

Ravi Kant Tiwari
MBBS, MD (Pharmacology)

Assistant Professor
Department of Pharmacology
Heritage Institute of Medical Sciences (HIMS)
Varanasi, UP

CBSPD

CBS Publishers & Distributors Pvt Ltd

New Delhi • Bengaluru • Chennai • Kochi • Kolkata • Lucknow • Mumbai
Hyderabad • Jharkhand • Nagpur • Patna • Pune • Uttarakhand

Understanding
Experimental Pharmacology

ISBN: 978-93-88108-44-7

First Edition: 2019

Reprint: 2023, 2024

Published by Satish Kumar Jain and Produced by Varun Jain for

CBS Publishers & Distributors Pvt Ltd

4819/XI Prahlad Street, 24 Ansari Road, Daryaganj, New Delhi 110 002, India
Ph: 011-23289259, 23266838   Website: www.cbspd.com
                                    e-mail: delhi@cbspd.com
Corporate Office: 204 FIE, Industrial Area, Patparganj, Delhi 110 092
Ph: 011-4934 4934   Fax: 011-4934 4935   e-mail: publishing@cbspd.com; publicity@cbspd.com

Branches

- **Bengaluru:** Seema House 2975, 17th Cross, K.R. Road, Banasankari 2nd Stage, Bengaluru 560 070, Karnataka, India
  Ph: +91-80-26771678/79   Fax: +91-80-26771680   e-mail: bangalore@cbspd.com
- **Chennai:** 7, Subbaraya Street, Shenoy Nagar, Chennai 600 030, Tamil Nadu, India
  Ph: +91-44-26680620, 26681266   Fax: +91-44-42032115   e-mail: chennai@cbspd.com
- **Kochi:** 42/1325, 1326, Power House Road, Opp KSEB, Power House, Ernakulam 682 018, Kerala, India
  Ph: +91-484-4059061-65   Fax: +91-484-4059065   e-mail: kochi@cbspd.com
- **Kolkata:** 147, Hind Ceramics Compound, 1st Floor, Nilgunj Road, Belghoria, Kolkata-700056 West Bengal, India
  Ph: 033-25633055, 033-25633056   e-mail: kolkata@cbspd.com
- **Lucknow:** Basement, Khushnuma Complex, 7-Meerabai Marg (Behind Jawahar Bhawan) Lucknow 226001, India
  Ph: 0522-4000032   e-mail: tiwari.lucknow@cbspd.com
- **Mumbai:** PWD Shed. Gala no. 25/26, Ramchandra Bhatt Marg, Next to JJ Hospital Gate no. 2, Opp. Union Bank of India Noorbaug Mumbai-400009, Maharashtra, India
  Ph: 022-66661880/89   e-mail: mumbai@cbspd.com

Representatives

- **Hyderabad**   0-9885175004   - **Jharkhand**   0-9811541605   - **Nagpur**   0-8692091830
- **Patna**   0-9334159340   - **Pune**   0-9664372571   - **Uttarakhand**   0-9716462459

Printed at Mudrak, Noida, UP, India

to

---

respected teachers
and
beloved students
of
pharmacology

Preface

Pharmacology is the essential basic medical subject. To understand the fundamentals and principles of pharmacology and therapeutics, a proper learning and understanding of the key concepts is necessary. This has given me the idea to write a book on practical aspects of experimental pharmacology. As a student, at both MBBS and MD levels, I always felt a need for a complete practical book in experimental pharmacology according to the curriculum. This book has been written to meet the demands of medical students not only for the examination purpose but also to give them the essential and fundamental concepts of pharmacology, especially pharmacodynamics through proper explanation of mechanism of action by experimental charts, graphs and practicals.

The experiments for teaching purpose are to be done on CAL as simulated experiments but still a proper and detailed explanation of the experimental procedure and methodology is required to understand the basic motive behind the experiment. This will help the students to correlate the concepts of pharmacodynamics with the pharmacotherapeutics. Suggestions for the improvement of this book are most welcome.

Ravi Kant Tiwari
drrkt1912@gmail.com

Acknowledgements

With an overwhelming sense of gratitude I have no words to express my deep regards to my revered teacher Prof (Dr) Priyamvada Sharma, Head, Department of Pharmacology, FH Medical College, Tundla, Firozabad (UP), for her inspiring guidance and motherly blessings. I am extremely grateful to Prof (Dr) PP Gupta, Head, Department of Pharmacology, AIIMS, Patna, for his encouragement through illuminating ideas, which I would remember throughout my life. I am deeply indebted to Prof (Dr) RK Goel, Head, Department of Pharmacology, Heritage Institute of Medical Sciences, Varanasi (UP), for having given me the opportunity to work under his able guidance. I am also very thankful to the faculty members of Department of Pharmacology, Heritage IMS, Varanasi, especially Dr Sandeep Kumar Gupta, Associate Professor, for their intellectual support and helpful discussions.

I am highly grateful to Dr Jamal Haider, Associate Professor, and Dr RP Yadav, Department of Pharmacology, BRD Medical College, Gorakhpur (UP), for guiding me throughout the preparation of the manuscript. I would like to give special thanks to Mr Anup Kumar, BRD Medical College, Gorakhpur, for nicely making the graphs of this manuscript.

I would like to thank all the medical colleagues, friends and students of pharmacology, who have been attached with my facebook page

Conceptual Pharmacology (www.conceptualpharmacology.com)

and for providing me the new ideas to be included in this book. I would like to give special thanks to the team of CBS Publishers and Distributors, New Delhi, for their continuous and timely support to publish this manuscript.

Ravi Kant Tiwari

Contents

1

Introduction to Experimental Pharmacology

PHARMACOLOGY

Branch of science, which deals with study of drugs on living systems.

EXPERIMENTAL PHARMACOLOGY

Study of effects of various pharmacological agents on different animal species.

- Originating in the 19th century, the discipline makes drug development possible.

- In the early 19th century, **Francois Magendie** (1809) studied the action of nux vomica (a strychnine containing plant) on dogs, and showed that spinal cord was its site of convulsant action.

- **Claude Bernard** (1842) discovered that the arrow poison curare acts at neuromuscular junction to block the neuromuscular transmission.

- **Rudolph Buchheim** (1847) is remembered for his pioneer work in experimental pharmacology.

- **Oswald Schmiedeberg** is considered as Father of Modern Pharmacology.

AIMS OF EXPERIMENTAL PHARMACOLOGY

1. Find out a therapeutic agent suitable for human use in preclinical studies.
2. Study the toxicity of a drug.
3. Study the mechanism and site of action of drug.

COMMON TERMINOLOGY

- *Ex vivo:* Outside the normal living organism (experiment on tissues from an organism in external environment).
- *In vitro:* Within glass usually in a cultured system.
- *In situ:* In biology and medical science, it means to examine the phenomenon exactly in place where it occurs (without moving it to some special medium).
- *In vivo:* Experiment on intact animal.
- *In silico/in silicio* (derived from silicon of computer chip): Performed on computer or via computer simulation.
- **The conventional teaching methods in experimental pharmacology involved the use of experimental instruments. Now the animal experiments for teaching purpose have shifted to simulation experiments on CAL (computer assisted learning).**

Experimental Animals

1. Rodents (mouse, rat, guinea pig).
2. Non-rodents (rabbit, monkey, dog, cat).
3. Others (frog, pigeon, zebra fish).

Rodents

1. **Mouse (*Mus musculus*):** Smallest lab animal. (Common strain = Swiss albino mice.) Easy to keep, handle and require small place for housing. There is large similarity in mice and human genome, therefore, they provide good model for study of mammalian biology and also for study on cancer, diabetes, immunological and autoimmune disorders, neurological, endocrine diseases. They are applied widely in acute toxicity studies and testing the drugs for teratogenicity.

- **Nude mice** = Hairless genetic mutant which lacks thymus gland.
- **Biege mice** = lack NK (natural killer) cells, susceptible to cancer.
- **Knockout mice** = Selective suppression of gene.
- **Knockin mice** = Selective introduction of gene.

2. **Rat (*Rattus norvegicus*)**
   - Most commonly used animal in biomedical research.
   - Albino rats
     - Wistar rats (wide head, long ear, small tail).
     - Sprague-Dawley rats (long and narrow head, longer tail).
   - Nude rats, similar to nude mice, lack a normal thymus and functionally mature T cells, hairless, used in immunological research.
   - Rats do not have tonsil and gall bladder. Tail helps in thermoregulation. Do not vomit (because of lack of vomiting centre and presence of strong sphincter between stomach and oesophagus). Rats are used in—research of behaviour, pharmacology, physiology, neuroscience, immunogenetics, cancer study, cardiovascular diseases, testing of psychopharmacological agents.
   - Study of drugs in acute and chronic BP effects.
   - Evaluation of antiulcer (gastric ulcer) drugs (Shay rat method of pyloric ligation).
   - Study of analgesic drugs on tail flick analgesiometer or Eddy's hot plate.
   - Acute and chronic toxicity studies.
   - Teratogenicity and carcinogenicity.

3. **Guinea pigs (*Cavia porcellus*)**
   - Herbivorous
   - Require vitamin C (ascorbic acid in food because unable to synthesise daily vitamin C requirement).
   - Guinea pigs are sensitive to many infections which make it suitable for the diagnostic tests.

- Ideal model for enteric amoebiasis, bronchial asthma, COPD and for screening of local anaesthetics.
- Susceptible for TB and anaphylactic shock, highly sensitive to histamine and penicillin.

Non-rodents

4. Rabbit (*Oryctolagus cuniculus*)

- Most common strain used in lab New Zealand white rabbit.
- Most suitable model for pyrogen testing of intravenous fluids.
- Other uses: Screening of diabetes, diphtheria, TB, cancer, heart diseases, genetics, nutrition, physiology, reproduction, and to test toxic effect of cosmetics and pharmaceuticals, good model for production of antibodies and antiserum.
- Very sensitive to histamine, ideal animal for PK (pharmacokinetic study).
- Enzyme atropine esterase is present in blood, which degrades atropine.

5. Monkey (*Macaca mulatta*)

- Rhesus monkey (large animal).
- Used as primate model to study drug metabolism because they show metabolic pattern similar to humans.
- Ideal model for PK study.
- Used for action of drugs on CNS (memory, anxiety, antidepressants, etc.), CVS (antianginal, antihypertensives, etc.), GIT and fertility.
- Require regular check up for rabies, TB and timely immunization.

6. Dog

- Small alimentary tract and easily get trained.
- Mongrel and beagle variety.
- Cardiovascular research, drugs acting on BP, vasomotor reversal phenomenon of Dale.
- Used as model for CVS research, diabetes mellitus, CNS, etc.

7. Cat
- Carnivorous, has nictitating membrane.
- Nictitating membrane is used in screening of ganglion blocking drugs.
- Used for behavioural studies, CNS studies, nerve impulse transmission, e.g. reflexes of respiratory system, spinal reflexes, and light perception.
- Also used in neuropharmacology.

8. Frog (*Rana tigrina*)
- Experiments on frogs are totally banned and they are endangered and protected species.
- Heart is three chambered (two atria, one ventricle).
- For CVS experiments or bioassay of acetylcholine on rectus abdominis muscle.
- Unlike in mammals where noradrenaline is the main neurotransmitter, in frog adrenaline is the main neurotransmitter in sympathetic system. Hence, frog heart is more sensitive to adrenaline.

As per guidelines of UGC (University Grants Commission) and MCI (Medical Council of India), the animal experiments are banned in India by dissection methods in undergraduate medical courses. Animal experiments are now replaced by computer models and simulation experiments (i.e. CAL).

Euthanasia

Humane killing (sacrifice) of an animal which produces rapid unconsciousness and subsequent death without or minimal pain or distress to animal.

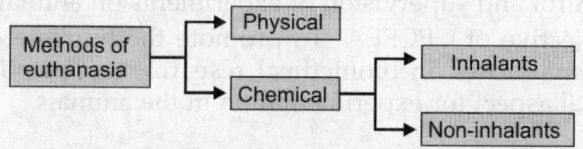

A. Physical methods: Performed by skilled, experienced personnel with appropriate, well-maintained equipment.
1. Cervical dislocation for rodents and small rabbits.
2. Decapitation for rodents and small rabbits.
3. Microwave irradiation.

B. Chemical methods:

1. Inhalant anaesthetics: Halothane, enflurane, sevo-flurane, methoxyflurane, isoflurane and desflurane.
   - Ether is not preferred now.
2. Non-inhalational anaesthetics:
   i. Barbiturates (sodium pentobarbital): IP (intra-peritoneal) in small animals, IV (intravenous) in non-rodents.
   ii. KCl: Induces immediate cardiac arrest without significant CNS depression, used after the animal is deeply anaesthetised.
   iii. $MgSO_4$: Causes cardiac arrhythmia, neuromuscular blockade and deep anaesthesia.
   iv. Neuromuscular blockers: For example, succinyl-choline induces muscular paralysis and death because of respiratory failure, but distress to the animal is more, hence less preferred.

Euthanasia in cold blooded (poikilothermic animal)

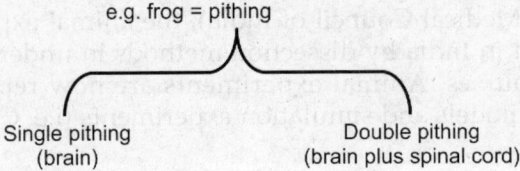

e.g. frog = pithing

Single pithing   Double pithing
(brain)   (brain plus spinal cord)

ANIMAL USE IN INDIA

- Supervised by **CPCSEA** (committee for the purpose of control and supervision of experiments on animals).
- Objective of CPCSEA: To promote the humane care of animals used in biomedical research and provide the legal aspect for experimentation in the animals.

Institutional Animal Ethics Committee: Members of IAEC

- A biological scientist.
- Two scientists from different biological disciplines.
- A veterinarian involved in care of animals.
- The scientist incharge of animal facility.

- A scientist from outside the institute.
- A socially aware non-scientific member.
- A representative or nominee of the CPCSEA.

KYMOGRAPH (SHERRINGTON–STARLING KYMOGRAPH) (Fig. 1.1)

It records contraction/relaxation movements of a tissue on moving surface.

- Used to obtain a graphical, amplified, measurable response of a muscle or tissue (contraction and relaxation), against a given concentration of drug or stimuli.
- It consists of the following parts:
1. **Motor box**: The important parts are:
   - **On/off switch** for power supply.
   - **Speed setting lever/variable speed lever**, to control the speed of clockwise rotating drum. The speed of drum depends on the type of tissue used.
   - **Clutch lever**, to disengage or engage the gear.
2. **Drum**: For most of the experiments, the speed of drum is kept at one revolution in 96 minutes.
3. **Spindle and screw**: Rod-like structure which holds the drum in the vertical position.

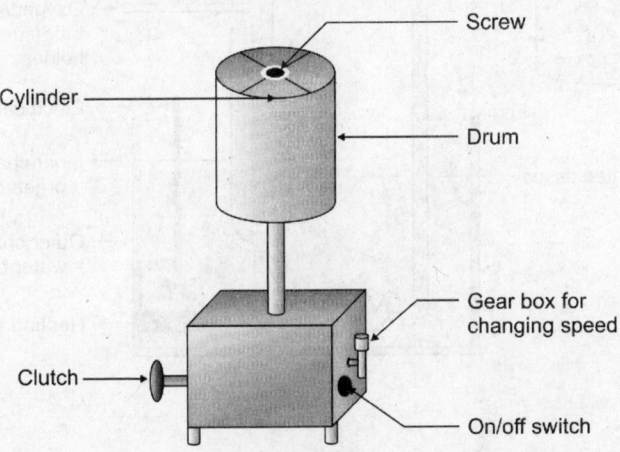

Fig. 1.1: Sherrington-Starling kymograph

- Height of the drum can be adjusted with lift screw attached at the top of the spindle.
- The kymograph paper (glossy surface out) is fixed tightly on the drum.
- Although smoking of kymograph paper is no more practiced due to health hazard, but can be performed where ink-writing device (pen) is unavailable at the tip of the lever.
- The drum is uniformly smoked with black soot (smoke) of benzene or kerosene or the mixture of the two.
- Uniform smoking is essential for proper recording.
- The recordings (tracings) on the smoked paper are preserved by properly fixing them with the help of fixing solution made of saturated solution of shellac and alcohol.
- No fixing is required for the ink-written tracings on the unsmoked paper.

Organ bath: **Rudolph Magnus** (1904) was the first to design the arrangement of bath for excised organs (Fig. 1.2).

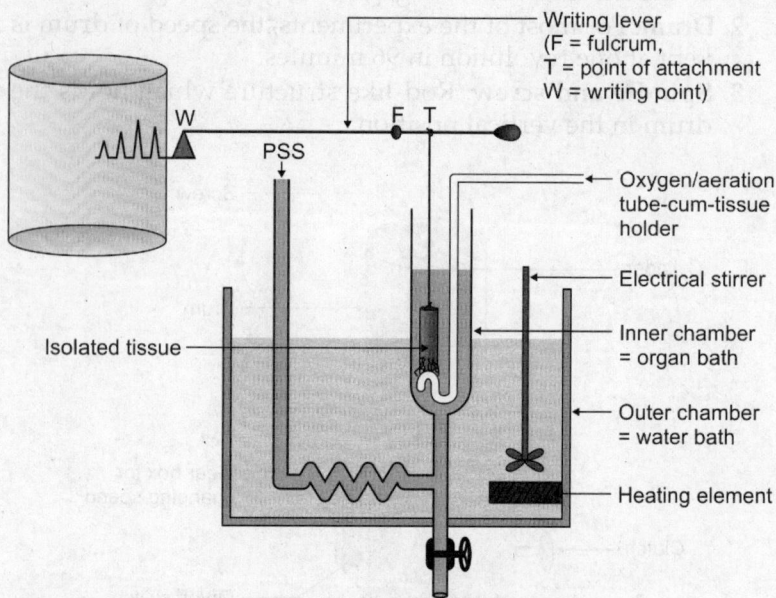

Fig. 1.2: Assembly of organ bath/student's organ bath for recording of contractions of isolated tissue (PSS = physiological salt solution)

The student organ bath consists of:

1. **A rectangular water bath or outer chamber**: Made of glass or perspex.
2. **A cylindrical organ bath or inner chamber**: Made of glass of variable capacity (5–100 ml) and filled with PSS (physiological salt-solution).
3. **Heating element and thermostat** in the outer chamber:
4. **Electrical stirrer in outer chamber**: To keep the water of outer chamber circulating for uniform heating.
5. **A glass coil at the lower end of inner chamber**: It ensures the warming of PSS before it enters in inner chamber.
6 **An oxygen tube-cum-tissue holder**: Made of glass, tissue is suspended through it in the PSS filled in inner chamber.
7. **A writing lever**
8. **Adjustable clamps and holders** for holding oxygen tube, writing lever and thermometer in position.

QUESTIONS

Q 1. **Comment on rat as experimental animal.**
Q 2. **Comment on CPCSEA.**
Q 3. **Comment on methods of euthanasia in experimental animals.**
Q 4. **Draw a set up of Sherrington kymograph with rotating drum and organ bath.**

2

General Instructions

1. KYMOGRAPH TRACING
It should be carefully prepared and should show: (a) Date, (b) experiment number, (c) type of preparation, (d) point of drug administration and (e) physiological fluid used.

2. USE OF DRUM
(i) It should be in the neutral gear when drum is not in use. (ii) The speed of drum for isolated tissue is slower than for heart experiment.

3. LIVING TISSUE
It must be handled with extreme care. (i) Stretching, crushing, drying or mishandling destroys the cells and proper responses may not be obtained. (ii) Oxygenation by aeration tube is essential for maintaining the respiration of isolated tissue. It also helps in proper mixing of the administered drugs. (iii) Maintenance of optimum temperature in bath (37–38°C) fluid is essential for mammalian (rabbit) isolated tissues (smooth muscles).

4. PHYSIOLOGICAL SOLUTIONS
- The tissues will survive only if they are bathed in a suitable solution. If wrong solution is used, the tissue responses are unreliable and survival is reduced. It is different for different tissues.

10

- **Physiological salt solution (PSS):** When animal experiment has to be done with isolated organ it is necessary to use certain type of physiological solution of different ionic concentrations which almost act as a substitute to their tissue fluid.
- They provide isotonicity, nutrition and act as buffer when drugs are added.
- It was Ringer who first introduced the idea that tissue could be kept alive by providing proper nutrition, O_2 and temperature.
- **Physiological salt solution can be defined as artificially prepared solution to keep isolated tissue alive under experiment condition. It should be prepared freshly and used within 24 hours.**

The compositions of commonly used physiological solutions are as follows:

A. Frog's Ringer solution

NaCl	6.5 gm
KCl	0.14 gm
$CaCl_2$	0.12 gm
$NaHCO_3$	0.20 gm
NaH_2PO_4	0.008 gm
Glucose	2.0 gm
Distilled water	1.0 litre

Note: (i) NaH_2PO_4 and glucose can be omitted for frog's Ringer's solution.

(ii) It is used for frog heart experiment and other isolated tissues of frog.

B. Ringer-Locke solution (mammalian Ringer solution)

NaCl	9.0 gm
KCl	0.42 gm
$CaCl_2$	0.25 gm
$NaHCO_3$	0.5 gm
Glucose	1.0–2.0 gm
Distilled water up to	1.0 litre

Note: It is aerated with oxygen or air and used for mammalian isolated heart and other tissues.

C. Tyrode solution

NaCl	8.0 gm
KCl	0.2 gm
NaHCO$_3$	1.0 gm
CaCl$_2$	0.2 gm
MgCl$_2$	0.01–0.1 gm
NaH$_2$PO$_4$	0.05 gm
Glucose	1.0 gm
Distilled water up to	1.0 litre

Note: It is used for rabbit and guinea pig intestine experiments.

Common ions and their significance are

- **Na$^+$:** Responsible for maintenance of isotonicity of muscle and nerve.
- **K$^+$:** Responsible for relaxation of heart, increases neuromuscular transmission and maintain the membrane potential of nerve.
- **Ca^{2+}:** Increases force of contraction, tone of heart and decreases excitability of nervous tissue.
- **Mg^{2+}:** Responsible for relaxation of smooth muscle.
- **pH:** 7.3–7.8 (at lower pH, tone of the tissue is decreased).
- **Glucose:** Serves as energy source and increases contractility of tissue.
- **Distilled water:** Acts as vehicle to dissolve various ingredients.
- **Temperature:** 37°–39°C. Maintenance of temperature is required in mammalian tissue, whereas the amphibian tissue survives at room temperature.
- **Aeration:** Air (O$_2$) + 5% CO$_2$ is needed for aeration. (Solution in the inner bath should be changed because it can alter the pH.)

Different PSS

1. **Ringer-Locke's solution (mammalian Ringer):** Isolated rabbit heart perfusion.
2. **Frog Ringer solution:** Frog heart experiment, frog rectus abdominis, leech dorsalis muscle preparation.

3. **Tyrode solution:** Rabbit intestine, guinea pig intestine (ileum).
4. **De Jalon's solution:** Rat uterus, duodenum and colon.
5. **Krebs-Henseleit solution:** Guinea pig tracheal chain. Rabbit aortic strip preparation.

Parameter to be Studied in a Curve/Graph Obtained (e.g. Rabbit/Guinea Pig Ileum Experiment)

1. **Frequency or rate:** Number of contraction per unit time, in the graph it is shown by distance between two waves.
2. **Amplitude:** Height of wave denotes force of contraction.
3. **Tone:** It is partially contracted state of muscle and elevated by stimulant and lowered by depressant. It is obtained by joining midpoint of 4–5 consecutive contractions which are equal in frequency, amplitude and tone.

Normal contraction: 3–4 contractions having same frequency, amplitude and tone.

Petri dish: It is used to keep isolated tissue in PSS while fixing the thread on both ends.

Lever

It is a device by which response of isolated tissue can be recorded and magnified.

- Made up of light aluminium, stainless steel. Most of levers are light in weight and fine but rigid as compared to their apparatus so that writing on smoked surface they do not lose their sensitivity (Fig. 2.1).

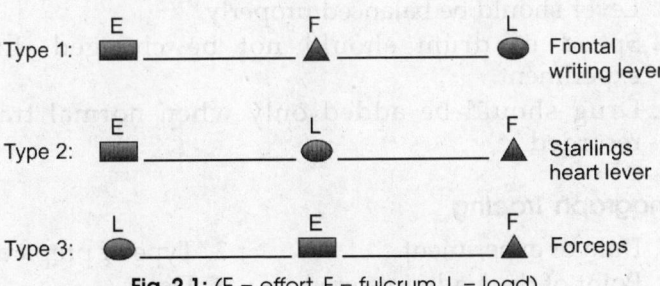

Fig. 2.1: (E = effort, F = fulcrum, L = load)

$$\text{Magnification } (Mx) = \frac{\text{Distance from F to L}}{\text{Distance from F to E}}$$

$$= \frac{FL}{FE}$$

Classification: On the basis of perpendicular, and tangential force and to give recording.

I. Tangent force:
  a. Simple lever which will give recording in curve line.
  b. Gimbal lever
  c. Torsion lever

II. Perpendicular force:
  a. Frontal writing lever
  b. Starling heart lever
  c. Auxotonic lever

- **Universal lever:** It is used for sudden repetitive contraction of muscle or movement, e.g. gastrocnemius muscle and sciatic nerve.
- **According to tension and length:** Two types
  1. Isotonic lever: Tension remains same, length altered, e.g. most of the levers.
  2. Isometric lever: Length remain same but force tension changed, e.g. auxotonic lever.

Precautions

1. Should not be overstretched.
2. Should be handled gently.
3. Bath temperature should be maintained at 37–38°C in warm-blooded animals.
4. Lever should be balanced properly.
5. Speed of drum should not be changed during experiment.
6. Drug should be added only when normal tracing recorded.

Kymograph Tracing

1. Date of experiment.
2. Type of preparation.
3. Point of drug administered.
4. Doses.

Purpose of Sensitivity Test

- To see the stability of preparation (qualitative assessment).
- To compare the drug effect from sensitivity (quantitative assessment).
- To see the effect of overnight fasting or any substance in meal that has altered gut response.

Error: Two types

Biological variation

    a. Downregulation of receptor due to overwashing of tissue.

    b. Animal used of different species of particular age and weight.

    c. Lab condition may vary.

    d. Faulty housing and handling of animal.

Methodological error

1. **Human error**
   a. Tissue selection and PSS preparation.
   b. Amount should be adequate.
2. **Experimental error**
   a. Proper balancing of lever.
   b. Maintaining temperature.

QUESTIONS

Q 1. What are the important precautions during experiment?

Q 2. Define PSS. Give the composition of frog Ringer solution. Mention its uses.

Q 3. Give the composition of Tyrode solution. Mention its uses.

Q 4. Name some PSS. Mention the importance of electrolytes present in them.

Q 5. What do you understand by lever and its magnification? Give some examples of lever.

Pharmacology of Receptors

- **Receptor**: A macromolecule, mostly protein, located on cell membrane or the cytosol or nucleus, to which a ligand binds.
- **Ligand**: A molecule that binds with receptor.
- **Affinity**: Binding capacity of ligand with the receptor.
- **Efficacy/intrinsic activity**: The subsequent events/responses produced by binding of the ligand with receptor. Depending on the affinity and intrinsic activity a ligand/drug can be:

Agonist
Antagonist
Partial agonist
Inverse agonist.

1. **Agonist**: It initiates the pharmacological action after binding with the receptor. Agonists have high affinity and high intrinsic activity (IA = 100% = 1), e.g. acetylcholine at muscarinic and nicotinic receptors, Morphine at mu opioid receptor.
2. **Antagonist**: It binds on the same site on the receptor, where the agonist binds but does not initiate any pharmacological action. So the antagonists have affinity but without intrinsic activity (IA = 0). They are simply blockers at the receptor site, e.g. atropine at muscarinic receptor, naloxone at mu opioid receptor.

3. **Partial agonist**: It has affinity equal to or less than the agonist and submaximal intrinsic activity (IA between 0 to + 1). Such drugs will not produce the full pharmacological response on the tissue. Partial agonist may also act as partial antagonist, because it occupies the receptors and minimize the number of vacant receptors to which the agonist bind.

4. **Inverse agonist:** It has affinity to the receptor but produces pharmacological actions opposite to that produced by agonist (IA = −1), e.g. beta-carbolines at benzodiazepine (BZD) binding sites of $GABA_A$ receptor. They produce actions opposite to that of BZDs (e.g. arousal and anxiety). Another important feature for inverse agonists is that, the receptor on which they bind show basal constitutive activity.

Upregulation and Downregulation of Receptors

Prolonged and administration of high concentration of antagonist result in increase in the number of receptors and/ or their externalization, the process is called upregulation of receptor. Similarly, the prolonged and administration of high concentration of agonist may result in decrease in the number of receptors or internalization of receptors, called downregulation of receptors.

Types of Receptors

1. G-protein coupled receptors (GPCRs)
2. Ligand gated ion channels (ionotropic receptors)
3. Enzyme linked receptors (protein kinase or tyrosine kinase)
4. Cytosolic or nuclear receptors affecting gene transcription.

Ligand Gated Ion Channels

- Located on cell membrane.
- Binding of agonist/drug results in depolarization or hyperpolarization of the cell.
- Nicotinic cholinergic receptors.
- $GABA_A$ receptor.
- Glycine receptor.

GPCRs

- G-proteins (guanine nucleotide binding proteins) are linked with these seven transmembrane (7-TM)/hepta-helical receptors.
- Three extracellular and three intracellular loops.
- Different types of G-proteins (Gs, Gi, Go, etc.) exist.
- Muscarinic cholinergic receptors.
- Alpha- and beta-adrenergic receptors.
- Dopaminergic receptors
- Serotonergic (5-HT) receptors (except 5-HT3).
- Most of the drugs act via GPCRs.

Enzyme-Linked Receptors

- Insulin
- Growth factors

Cytosolic or Nuclear Receptors Affecting Gene Transcription

- Steroidal hormones
- Thyroid hormones
- PPAR (peroxisome proliferator activated receptor)
- Retinoid receptor

Spare receptors/Receptor reserve: Maximum pharmacological response can be achieved by a drug even when less than 100% of the receptors are occupied by the drug. These unoccupied extra receptors are called spare receptors/receptor reserve.

Silent receptor: Plasma proteins (albumin) to which drugs bind but does not elicit any pharmacological action or effect.

Orphan receptor: Receptors for which no endogenous ligand exist.

QUESTION

Q 1. **Compare and contrast**
   a. **Agonist, antagonist, inverse agonist and partial agonist.**
   b. **GPCR and ligand-gated ion channel.**
   c. **Silent and orphan receptors.**
   d. **Upregulation and downregulation of receptor.**

4

Cholinergic and Adrenergic System, Receptors and Drugs

INTRODUCTION

Autonomic nervous system consists of two divisions—parasympathetic (rest and digest actions) and sympathetic system (fight, flight or fright actions).

Neurotransmitters in ANS

1. At all the ganglionic synapse of ANS (whether sympathetic or parasympathetic) → acetylcholine.
2. All postganglionic parasympathetic fibres → acetylcholine.
3. Most of postganglionic sympathetic fibres → norepinephrine.

Points to Remember

a. Postganglionic sympathetic fibres to sweat glands → acetylcholine.
b. Postganglionic sympathetic fibres at splanchnic and renal blood vessels → dopamine.
c. The chromaffin cells of adrenal medulla are innervated by preganglionic sympathetic neurons, where the neurotransmitter is acetylcholine. On stimulation, these cells predominantly secrete epinephrine with a small amount of norepinephrine.

Cholinergic Transmission

1. Synthesis of the transmitter (acetylcholine)
2. Storage
3. Release
4. Termination of action of released transmitter.
   - Choline uptake (rate limiting step in biosynthesis of acetylcholine) is blocked by hemicholinium.
   - Vesicular transport of acetylcholine into storage vesicles is blocked by vesamicol.
   - Botulinum toxin interferes with the exocytotic release of acetylcholine.
   - Cholinesterase is the enzyme responsible for hydrolyzing the released acetylcholine into choline and acetate, which are recycled for ACh synthesis.
     a. True cholinesterase/acetylcholinesterase
     b. Pseudocholinesterase/butyrylcholinesterase

Cholinergic Receptors/Cholinoceptors

1. **Muscarinic (GPCRs): M1–M5.**
2. **Nicotinic (ligand-gated ion channels): N_M, N_N.**
   - **M1 muscarinic receptor**: At autonomic ganglia, gastric glands and CNS. Gq protein coupled, responsible for learning and memory, and gastric acid secretion.
   - **M2 muscarinic receptor**: At cardiac muscle and visceral smooth muscles, also in CNS. Gi/Go protein coupled, responsible for negative chronotropic, inotropic and dromotropic action (reduced heart rate, reduced force of cardiac contraction and reduced conduction velocity in cardiac tissues), and contraction in visceral smooth muscles.
   - **M3 muscarinic receptor:** At visceral smooth muscles, iris smooth muscles (circular = sphincter pupillae), ciliary muscle of eye, exocrine glands and vascular endothelium. Gq protein coupled, responsible for contraction of smooth muscles, miosis (pupillary constriction), spasm of accommodation, glandular secretion and vasodilatation through release of NO (= EDRF).

- **M4, M5 muscarinic receptors:** At nerve endings in CNS and regulate the release of other neurotransmitters.
- **N_M Nicotinic receptors:** At skeletal muscle motor end plate (= neuromuscular junction), responsible for contraction of skeletal muscle.
- **N_N Nicotinic receptors:** At autonomic ganglia (both sympathetic and parasympathetic), adrenal medulla and CNS, responsible for transmission of impulse through autonomic ganglia, release of catecholamines from adrenal medulla and excitation/inhibition in CNS.

CLASSIFICATION OF CHOLINOMIMETICS

1. **Directly acting:** Acetylcholine, methacholine, carbachol, bethanechol, pilocarpine.
2. **Indirectly acting (anticholinesterases):**
   a. Reversible: Physostigmine, neostigmine, pyridostigmine, rivastigmine, edrophonium, ambenonium, demecarium, donepezil.
   b. Irreversible: Malathion, parathion, diazinon, ecothiophate, isoflurophate, propoxur, tabun, sarin, soman.

PHARMACOLOGICAL ACTIONS OF CHOLINOMIMETICS

Muscarinic Actions

1. **Eye:** Miosis (Pupillary constriction), spasm of accommodation and reduced IOP = M3 action
2. **Lungs:** Bronchoconstriction and increased bronchial secretion = M3 action
3. **CVS:** Decreased (HR, force of cardiac contraction, and conduction velocity) = M2 action. Fall of BP (hypotension, due to vasodilatation produced by EDRF/NO, released from endothelium of blood vessels) = M3 action.
4. **Sweat glands and salivary glands:** Increased secretions = M3 action.
5. **GIT:** Gastric acid secretion = M1 action. Increased GI motility (tone of GIT muscles increased with relaxation of sphincters) and increased GIT secretion = M3 action.

6. **Urinary bladder:** Contraction of detrusor muscle and relaxation of sphincter (voiding of urine) = M3 action.
7. **Male sex organs:** Erection of penis = M3 action through the release of NO/EDRF. (Ejaculation is a sympathetic response = α_1 action)

Nicotinic Actions

1. **Autonomic ganglia:** Stimulation of sympathetic and parasympathetic ganglia, and release of catecholamines or ACh from postganglionic sites, release of adrenaline from adrenal medulla = N_N action.
2. This is the basis of nicotinic/ganglionic action of high dose of acetylcholine given after atropine (manifested as rise of BP and tachycardia).
3. **Skeletal muscle:** Fasciculations followed by paralysis due to persistent depolarization = N_M action.

CNS Actions (Muscarinic and Nicotinic)

Complex actions, CNS stimulation (tremors, convulsions, behavioral disturbances) followed by depression of CNS.

INDIVIDUAL AGENTS

- **Acetylcholine:** Not used clinically because of non-selective and very short duration of action.
- **Methacholine:** Obsolete now.
- **Carbachol:** Marked nicotinic actions.
- **Bethanechol:** Has muscarinic actions, used to reverse postoperative atony of urinary bladder, and to combat urinary retention due to non-obstructive causes. Also used to treat GI atony.
- **Pilocarpine:** Tertiary amine, used as eyedrops in the treatment of glaucoma (third line drug), and to counteract mydriatics because being a cholinomimetic, it produces miosis.
- **Physostigmine:** Ophthalmic uses has declined now. A tertiary amine, lipid soluble, crosses BBB, can be used as antidote of belladonna/atropine poisoning.

- **Neostigmine:** Quaternary compound, lipid insoluble, does not cross BBB, used in the treatment of myasthenia gravis, paralytic ileus, and atony of urinary bladder and postoperative decurarization.
- **Pyridostigmine:** In the treatment of myasthenia gravis.
- **Edrophonium:** In diagnosing myasthenia gravis.
- **Rivastigmine:** In the treatment of Alzheimer's disease.
- **Donepezil:** In the treatment of Alzheimer's disease.
- **Organophosphorus compounds (irreversible anticholinesterases):** No therapeutic use, only of toxological importance.

ANTICHOLINERGICS

A. **Antimuscarinic:** Atropine and atropine-like drugs.

B. **Antinicotinic:** Neuromuscular (N_M) blockers and ganglion (N_N) blockers.

ANTIMUSCARINIC DRUGS

- **Scopolamine:** Motion sickness, narcoanalysis.
- **Trihexyphenidyl/benzhexol:** Parkinson's disease.
- **Tropicamide:** Mydriatic.
- **Homatropine:** Mydriatic.
- **Cyclopentolate:** Mydriatic.
- **Ipratropium:** COPD, bronchial asthma.
- **Tiotropium:** COPD, bronchial asthma.
- **Atropine:** Preanesthetic medication.
- **Glycopyrrolate:** Preanaesthetic medication.
- **Pirenzepine:** Peptic ulcer.
- **Telenzepine:** Peptic ulcer.
- **Dicyclomine:** Antispasmodic, colicky pain.
- **Clidinium bromide:** Antispasmodic, colicky pain, IBS.
- **Oxybutynin:** Nocturnal enuresis, urinary frequency, urge incontinence, neurogenic bladder.
- **Tolterodine:** Urinary frequency, urge incontinence, neurogenic bladder.
- **Drotaverine:** Non-antimuscarinic antispasmodic, PDE-4 inhibitor, intestinal, biliary, renal colic and uterine colic.
- **Flavoxate:** Urinary frequency, urge incontinence, neurogenic bladder.

- **Valethamate:** Intestinal, biliary, renal colic and uterine colic, and for dilatation of cervix.

Pharmacological Actions of Atropine (Prototype of Antimuscarinics): Non-selective muscarinic antagonist.
1. **Eye:** Passive mydriasis, abolition of light reflex, cycloplegia and increased IOP.
2. **CVS:** Tachycardia, without any consistent effect on BP.
3. **Smooth muscles:** Relaxation, tone of GIT is reduced, bronchodilatation.
4. **Glands:** Decreases secretion.
5. **CNS:** Stimulant action followed by CNS depression at higher dose.
6. **Miscellaneous:** Rise of body temperature.

Catecholamines

The sympathomimetic amines having hydroxyl (OH^-) substitution at 3,4-position of benzene ring (= catechol nucleus) are called catecholamines.
1. Endogenous: Dopamine, noradrenaline, adrenaline.
2. Exogenous: Dobutamine, isoprenaline.

Endogenous Catecholamines

- Norepinephrine (NE) is the principal transmitter of most sympathetic postganglionic fibers and of certain tracts in the CNS.
- Dopamine (DA) is the predominant transmitter of the mammalian extrapyramidal system and of several mesocortical and mesolimbic neuronal pathways.
- Epinephrine (EPI) is the major hormone of the adrenal medulla.
- Collectively, these three amines are called *catecholamines.*

Adrenergic Transmission

Steps

1. Synthesis of catecholamines.
2. Storage of catecholamines.

3. Release of catecholamines.
4. Reuptake and termination of action of catecholamines.
5. Metabolism of catecholamines.

Prejunctional regulation of norepinephrine release

- The release of the three sympathetic cotransmitters can be modulated by prejunctional autoreceptors and hetero-receptors.
- Following their release from sympathetic terminals, all three cotransmitters—NE, NPY, and ATP—can feedback on prejunctional receptors to inhibit the release of each other.
- The most thoroughly studied have been prejunctional α_2 adrenergic receptors.
- The α_2 adrenergic receptors are the principal prejunctional receptors that inhibit sympathetic neurotransmitter release.
- Antagonists of α_2 adrenergic receptors, in turn, can enhance the release of sympathetic neurotransmitter.

Activation of numerous heteroreceptors on sympathetic nerve varicosities can inhibit the release of sympathetic neurotransmitters; these include

- M2 and M4 muscarinic
- 5HT
- PGE2
- Histamine
- Enkephalin and
- DA receptors.

Enhancement of sympathetic neurotransmitter release can be produced by activation of:

- β_2 adrenergic receptors,
- Angiotensin AT2 receptors, and
- Nicotinic acetylcholine receptors

METABOLISM OF CATECHOLAMINES

- Following uptake, catecholamines can be metabolized (in neuronal and nonneuronal cells) or re-stored in vesicles (in neurons).

- Two enzymes are important in the initial steps of metabolic transformation of catecholamines—MAO and COMT.

Adrenergic Receptors

- Ahlquist (1948) proposed the existence of more than one adrenergic receptor.
- Adrenergic receptors are broadly classified as either α, β and D with subtypes within each group.
- Adrenergic receptors are GPCRs.
- α_1: α_1A, α_1B, α_1D.
- α_2: α_2A, α_2B, α_2C.
- β_1
- β_2
- β_3
- D1 (D1 and D5).
- D2 (D2, D3, D4).

Classification of Sympathomimetics

Catecholamines and sympathomimetic drugs are classified as

- *Direct acting*
- *Indirect-acting (amphetamine, tyramine)*
- *Mixed-acting sympathomimetics (ephedrine).*

Adrenergic Agonists

Direct Acting:
1. Selective:
    - α_1: Phenylephrine
    - α_2: Clonidine
    - β_1: Dobutamine
    - β_2: Terbutaline
2. Nonselective
    - $\alpha_1 \alpha_2$: Oxymetazoline
    - $\beta_1 \beta_2$: Isoprenaline
    - $\alpha_1 \alpha_2 \beta_1 \beta_2$: Adrenaline
    - $\alpha_1 \alpha_2 \beta_1$: Noradrenaline

Mixed Acting

Ephedrine (α_1 α_2 β_1 β_2), and releasing agent.

Indirect Acting

- Releasing agents: Amphetamine, tyramine
- Uptake inhibitor: Cocaine
- MAO inhibitors: Selegiline
- COMT inhibitors: Entacapone

ADRENERGIC DRUGS AND RECEPTORS

- Adrenaline (epinephrine): α_1, α_2, β_1, β_2, weak β_3
- Noradrenaline (norepinephrine, levarterenol): α_1, α_2, β_1, $\beta3$
- Isoprenaline (isoproterenol): β_1, β_2, β_3
- Dopamine: D1, D2, β_1, α
- Dobutamine: β_1, α
- Fenoldopam: D1
- Dopexamine: D1, D2, β_2
- Ephedrine: α, β
- Amphetamine: α, β
- Oxymetazoline: α_1, α_2
- Phenylephrine: α_1
- Methoxamine: α_1
- Clonidine: α_2
- Apraclonidine: α_2
- Salbutamol (albuterol): β_2

Cardiovascular Actions of Adrenaline

- The principal catecholamine (80–90%) secretion from adrenal medulla.
- The relative receptor affinity: ($\beta_2 > \beta_1 = \alpha_1 = \alpha_2$)
- At low doses β effects predominate over α effects.
- α effects are stronger at high doses.
- It also has weak β_3 agonist action.

When Administered by SC Injection or Slow IV Infusion

1. Adrenaline increases systolic BP due to rise of peripheral vascular resistance due to vasoconstriction (α_1 action,

predominant action), and increased cardiac output due to rise of HR = positive chronotropic action (β_1 action) and increased force of contraction = positive inotropic action (β_1 action).
2. Adrenaline decreases diastolic BP (β_2 action).
3. The mean BP increases slightly. (Mean BP = DBP + 1/3rd PP).

When Administered by Rapid IV Injection

- Both SBP and DBP increases (α_1 effect predominate). (SBP>DBP, and PP increases).
- After a few minutes BP comes to normal followed by secondary fall in MBP before coming to normal. (Due to fall in concentration of adrenaline, now β_2 effect is seen, i.e. vasodilatation.)

Adrenaline Administered in Low Doses

Produces fall in diastolic BP due to reduced peripheral resistance because of vasodilatation (it is due to greater sensitivity of β_2 receptors as compared to α receptors at low doses).

Vasomotor Reversal of Dale

- Prior administration of alpha-blocker will produce only fall of BP, due to β_2 effect.
- Pressor response (biphasic response) of adrenaline is converted to a depressor response.

CARDIOVASCULAR ACTIONS OF NORADRENALINE

- ($\alpha_1 = \alpha_2 > \beta_1 >> \beta_2$)
- Increases both SBP and DBP.
- Reflex bradycardia is seen (due to compensatory increase in vagal discharge), this is secondary to hypertension produced by noradrenaline.
- If atropine (which blocks the transmission of vagal effects) is given prior to noradrenaline, hypertension is followed by tachycardia.
- Dale's vasomotor reversal phenomenon is not seen with noradrenaline (unlike adrenaline, it has very little β_2 action).

CARDIOVASCULAR ACTIONS OF ISOPRENALINE

- It has a predominant β_1 and β_2, weak β_3 and negligible α action.
- ($\beta_1 = \beta_2 >> \beta_3 >>>> \alpha$)
- Positive inotropic and chronotropic effect on heart causing increase in cardiac output (β_1 effect).
- Slight increase in SBP.
- DBP is greatly reduced (because of β_2 effect, leading to fall of peripheral vascular resistance).
- Mean BP is reduced.
- Tachycardia.

DOPAMINE

- Endogenous catecholamine, immediate precursor of noradrenaline.
- Agonist at D1, D2, β_1 and α receptors, but not on β_2.
- At low doses, infusion rate of 2–5 microgram/kg/min, it stimulates dopamine D1 receptors of renal and mesenteric blood vessels, leading to vasodilatation in these blood vessels, increased GFR, and RBF.
- This effect is valuable in patients of hypovolaemic shock.
- As the rate of infusion is increased to 5–10 microgram/kg/min, it stimulates β_1 receptors, causing positive inotropic and weak chronotropic effect on heart.
- Further increase in concentration (10–20 microgram/kg/min or more), stimulates α receptors, increasing peripheral resistance and rise in BP.
- Dopamine does not cross BBB, so no CNS effects are produced on peripheral administration (not useful in Parkinson's disease).
- Metabolized by both MAO and COMT.

Indications

1. Shock: Cardiogenic shock, resulting from MI, trauma or surgery.

- Shock is a condition of low cardiac output with compromised renal perfusion.

- Hypovolaemia, if present, should be corrected with IV fluids.

2. Cardiac failure with oliguria: Dopamine is used for emergency treatment of cardiac failure due to its positive inotropic property (though dobutamine is a more selective inotropic agent, and preferred), however, DA is a drug of choice if cardiac failure is associated with oliguria.

Dobutamine

- Structural analogue of isoprenaline.

- Direct acting synthetic catecholamine.

- Dobutamine is a racemic mixture of (+) and (−) enantiomers.

- The (−) enantiomer acts as α_1 agonist, and increases vascular resistance, while the (+) enantiomer acts as potent β_1 agonist, weak β_2 agonist, and a potent α_1 antagonist [that block the effect of the (−) dobutamine].

- Thus dobutamine is a relatively selective β_1 agonist, with weak β_2 agonist action.

- Its major effect is increased myocardial contractility (β_1 effect) = positive inotropic effect, leading to increase in cardiac output.

- Very less chronotropic effect and change in peripheral resistance or BP, at usual infusion rate.

- It has no action on dopaminergic receptors, so no direct renal vasodilator effect, however, RBF increases with dobutamine as the CO increases.

- Dobutamine: Half life = 2 min, given by IV infusion (5–10 microgram/kg/min).

- Advantage of dobutamine over isoprenaline: Lesser chronotropic effect.

- Advantage of dobutamine over dopamine: Lesser peripheral vasoconstrictor effect.

- Indications of dobutamine:
  1. Short-term management of systolic heart failure with low output.
  2. Cardiogenic shock.
  3. Non-invasive assessment of coronary disease: Dobutamine stress echocardiography.

PHENYLEPHRINE

- α_1 selective agonist.
- Due to vasoconstriction, rise of BP is seen, accompanied by bradycardia.
- Active mydriasis (due to contraction of radial muscles of iris), without cycloplegia.
- IOT is reduced due to constriction of blood vessels of ciliary body.
- Used orally/topically as nasal decongestant, due to vasoconstriction of nasal mucosa through α_1 receptors present on venules.

Also used
- To control local bleeding (1%).
- As vasopressor agent (IM, SC or IV) to raise BP in hypotension due to sympathetic dysfunction (spinal injury/spinal anaesthesia).
- With local anaesthetic (1:20,000), to prolong the action and reduce the systemic side effects.

Anti-adrenergic Drugs

Anti-adrenergic drugs are classified into two groups:
  1. α blockers (α adrenergic receptor antagonists).
  2. β blockers (β adrenergic receptor antagonists).

Adrenergic neuron blockers

- They act by interfering with the storage or release of adrenergic transmitter on nerve stimulation.
- They reduce the delivery of catecholamine neurotransmitters to the adrenergic receptors.

- **Peripherally acting adrenergic neuron blockers:** *Guanethidine, Guanadrel.*
- **Peripherally as well as centrally acting adrenergic neuron blockers:** *Reserpine.*
- *Due to their prominent adverse effects and availability of better drugs, these drugs are not used now.*

Classification of Alpha Blockers

Nonselective
- Reversible: Phentolamine, tolazoline.
- Irreversible: Phenoxybenzamine.

Selective
- α_1 blockers: Prazosin, terazosin, doxazosin, alfuzosin, bunazosin, tamsulosin, silodosin.
- α_2 blockers: Yohimbine, idazoxan.

Miscellaneous
- Ergot alkaloids: Ergotamine, dihydroergotamine, ergotoxine, dihydroergotoxine.
- Chlorpromazine.

Beta Blockers

1. **First generation, nonselective β blockers:**
   - Propranolol
   - Nadolol
   - Sotalol
   - Timolol
2. **First generation, nonselective β blockers with ISA (intrinsic sympathomimetic activity)**
   - Pindolol
   - Oxprenolol
3. **Second generation, selective β_1 blockers**
   - Atenolol
   - Acebutalol
   - Bisoprolol
   - Esmolol
   - Metoprolol

4. **Third generation β blockers, with additional properties:**
   A. **Nonselective β blockers with additional property (α-blocking property)**
      - Labetalol
      - Carvedilol
   B. **Selective β_1 blockers with additional property (vasodilator property)**
      - Betaxolol
      - Celiprolol
      - Nebivolol

PHARMACOLOGICAL ACTIONS: PROPRANOLOL AS PROTOTYPE OF β BLOCKERS

Cardiovascular Effects

1. **Heart (blockade of β_1 receptors)**
   - Decreases HR.
   - Decreases force of contraction.
   - Decreases cardiac output.
   - Decreased conduction velocity.
   - Decreased workload by heart.
   - Decreased myocardial oxygen demand.
   - Decreased automaticity.
   - The response depends on degree of sympathetic activity, no significant effect at rest in normal individuals).
   - Propranolol has direct cardiac depressant (quinidine like) and membrane stabilizing action (local anaesthetic type), but little antiarrhythmic effect at usual doses.

2. **Blood vessels**
   - TPR is increased initially (due to blockade of β_2 receptor mediated vasodilatation) and CO is reduced (β_1 blockade).
   - So, little acute change in BP.

- But on prolonged administration BP gradually falls in hypertensives, not in normotensives.
- Because, after continued treatment resistance vessels adapt to chronically reduced CO and TPR decreases = BP decreases.

Antihypertensive mechanism of beta blockers
- Decreased cardiac output (blockade of β_1 receptors)
- Decreased TPR (after prolonged use)
- Decreased renin release from kidney (blockade of β_1 receptors)
- Reduced release of NE from sympathetic nerve terminals (blockade of β_1 presynaptic receptors, which facilitate NE release)
- Reduced central sympathetic outflow.

3. **Respiratory tract**
- In asthmatics, nonselective β blockers (propranolol) can cause severe bronchoconstriction (due to blocakde of β_2 receptors on bronchial smooth muscles, which are responsible for bronchodilation).
- The risk is less with cardioselective (β_1 selective) blockers.

4. **CNS actions**
- Lipid soluble agents cross CNS, produce sedation, disturbed sleep. Propranolol reduces anxiety for short-term basis, but this is not due to central (CNS) action.

5. **Ocular actions**
- Reduced aqueous humour formation, used in medical treatment of open angle glaucoma (timolol, levo-bunalol, betaxolol, carteolol).

6. **Miscellaneous actions**
- **Metabolic:** Delays recovery from hypoglycaemia, in patients of diabetes mellitus on insulin or OHAs, due to blockade of β_2 receptors in liver (= blockade of glycogenolysis). **Both nonselective (β_1, β_2) and cardio-selective (β_1) blockers, mask the warning signs (tachycardia) of hypoglycaemia in patients of DM.
- **Local anaesthetic:** Propranolol has this effect but not clinically used for this purpose, because it causes irritation at injection site.

- **Skeletal muscle:** Propranolol inhibits sympathetically induced tremor (benign or essential). This is due to peripheral action, directly on muscle fibres (through β_2 receptors).

Cardioselective β-Blockers

- Selective β_1 blockers.
- They block β_1 receptors at low and therapeutic dose, but can block β_2 receptors at higher dose.
- Cardioselectivity is relative and lost at higher doses.
- Atenolol
- Acebutalol
- Bisoprolol
- Esmolol
- Metoprolol
- Betaxolol
- Celiprolol
- Nebivolol

Beta Blockers with Intrinsic Sympathomimetic Activity (ISA)

ISA is due to their partial agonistic activity at β_1 or β_2 receptors, thus they cause submaximal stimulation of these receptors.

1. **Nonselectve:** Pindolol, oxprenolol
2. **β_1 selective:** Acebutalol, celiprolol

Mixed Alpha and Beta Blockers

- **Carvedilol**
- **Labetalol**
- **Bucindolol**
- **The alpha antagonist action contributes to vasodilatation, reducing PVR and results in fall of BP.**

Third Generation Beta Blockers with Vasodilator Property

- **Alpha and beta blockers**: Labetalol, carvedilol, bucindolol.

- **Beta blockers with nitric oxide (NO) production:** Nebivolol, celiprolol.
- **Beta blockers with calcium channel blocking action:** Carvedilol, betaxolol.
- **Beta blockers with antioxidant action:** Carvedilol.

QUESTIONS

Q 1. Classify cholinomimetics.

Q 2. Classify anticholinergics.

Q 3. Classify sympathomimetics.

Q 4. Classify sympatholytics.

Q 5. Comment on cardioselective beta blockers.

Q 6. Comment on third generation beta blockers.

Q 7. Comment on cholinergic and adrenergic receptors.

Q 8. Compare and contrast
   a. Dopamine and dobutamine
   b. Adrenaline and noradrenaline
   c. Adrenaline and ephedrine
   d. Phenoxybenzamine and prazosin
   e. Active and passive miosis
   f. Active and passive mydriasis

5

Dose Response Curve

- Pharmacodynamics deals with:

  1. The biological effects produced by drugs.

  2. Mechanism of action and site of action of drugs.

  3. The relationship between the plasma concentration of drug with its response and duration of action.

  4. ADRs (adverse drug reactions).

- In short, pharmacodynamics deals with what a drug does to the body.

Measurement of drug effects =
Quantitative aspects of drug effects

Dose Response Curve (DRC)

1. Graded dose response curves.

2. Quantal dose response curves.

1. Graded DRC: The graded dose response curves are obtained by administering increasing dose of the drug to a single subject or to an isolated tissue (Fig. 5.1a, b).

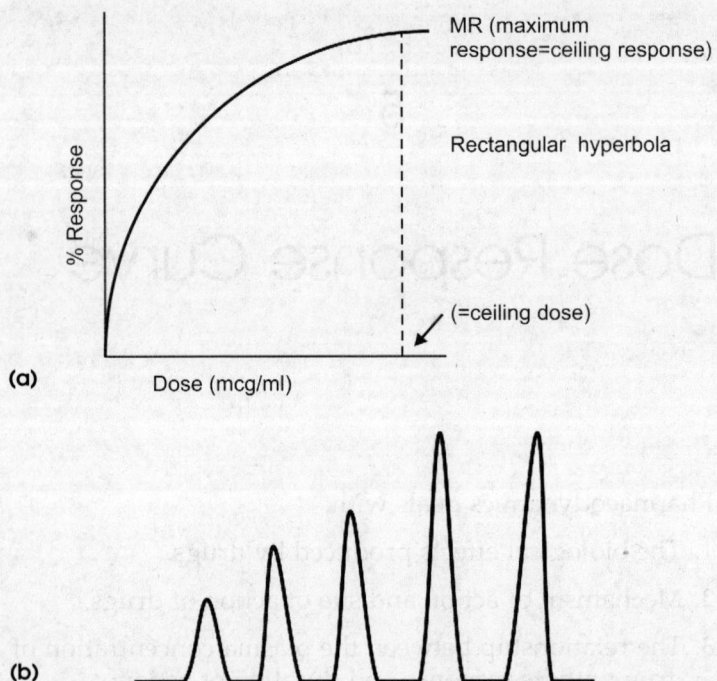

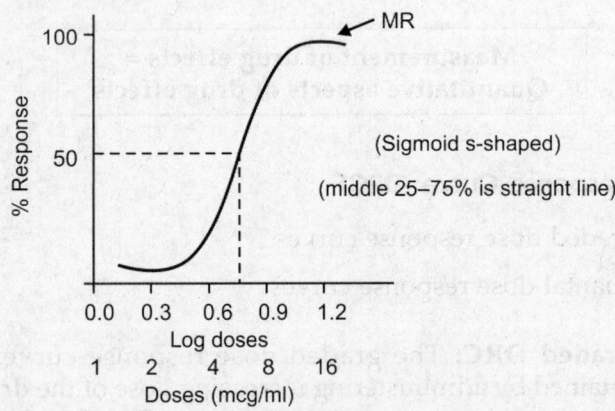

Fig. 5.1: (a) Dose response curve, **(b)** Ascending dose response plot.

Log Dose Response Curve (Fig. 5.2)

Fig. 5.2: Log dose response curve

Information derived from log dose response curve (Figs 5.3 and 5.4):

1. **ED_{50}:** From the middle portion (straight line) of the curve, we can find out ED_{50} of the drug.
   - ED_{50} means effective dose which can provide 50% of the maximal response.
   - Smaller the ED_{50}, more potent is the drug.
2. If two drugs produce same effects by the same mechanism, LDR (log dose response) curves of both drugs run parallel to each other and the LDR curve of less potent drug would be located on the right side on dose axis.
   - Look at X-axis
   - Potency (A) > (B), (Right shift of DRC = less potent).
3. **Potency:** Dose of drug required to produce a standard effect (closer the LDR curve towards y-axis, smaller is the dose required to produce the given effect, and hence greater the potency). [Potency decides dose selection.]

Efficacy: Maximum response, reflected by height of LDR curve on y-axis (response axis).

(Efficacy is more important than potency in drug selection)

In Fig. 5.3
   - Drug (A) and drug (B) have equal efficacy.

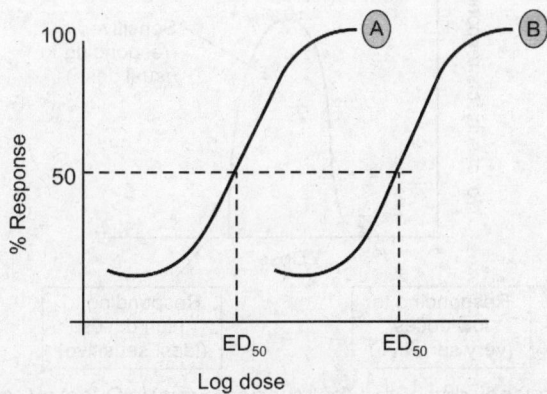

Fig. 5.3: Drugs (A) and (B) with similar efficacy but different potency

In Fig. 5.4

Potency (A) > (B) > (C) > (D)

Efficacy (B) = (C) > (A) > (D).

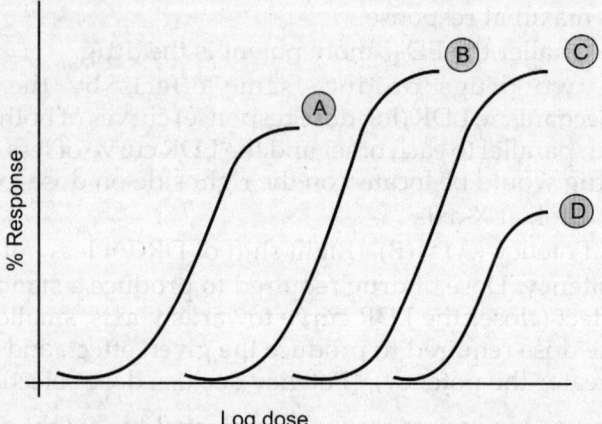

Fig. 5.4: Drugs (A), (B), (C) and (D) with their efficacy and potency

2. Quantal Dose Response Curves: All or none response (Bell-shaped DRC) (Fig. 5.5)

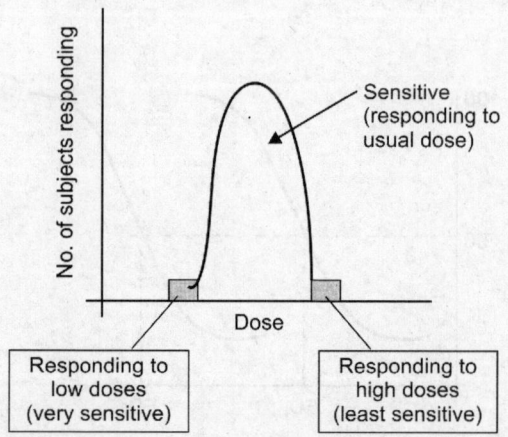

Fig. 5.5: Frequency distribution (bell-shaped curve) in Quantal (=all or none) response.

Pharmacological (= pharmacodynamic) antagonism

1. Competitive antagonism: Antagonist competes with the agonist for its binding sites on the receptor.
2. Noncompetitive antagonism: Antagonist antagonises the effect of agonist by acting at a site which is different from agonist receptor site (= allosteric antagonism).

1. **Reversible competitive (= equilibrium) antagonism:** Antagonist binds reversibly (by forming weak bonds) to the same receptor site as that of agonist. Hence the antagonism can be overcome (= surmountable) and the maximum response of agonist can be attained if the concentration of agonist is increased. Conversely, if the dose of antagonist is increased, the amount of agonist required to produce the maximal response would be greater, so ED_{50} of agonist in the presence of antagonist increases. Log dose response curve (LDRC) shows a parallel right shift, e.g. atropine is competitive antagonist for acetylcholine at muscarinic receptors. Propranolol is competitive antagonist for adrenaline, at β adrenergic receptors. Naloxone is competitive antagonist at μ opioid receptors for morphine (Fig. 5.6).

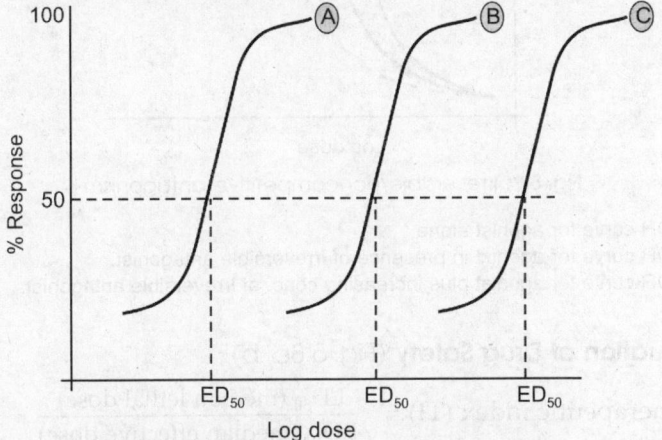

Fig. 5.6: Reversible competitive antagonism

A. LDR curve for agonist alone.
B. LDR curve for agonist in presence of competitive antagonist.
C. LDR curve for agonist plus increasing concentration of competitive antagonist.

2. **Irreversible (= nonequilibrium) antagonism** (Fig. 5.7):
   - Antagonist binds irreversibly forming a stable covalent bond to the same receptor site as for agonist.
   - Antagonism cannot be overcome (insurmountable) even by increasing the concentration of agonist.
   - Log dose response curve (LDRC) of agonist—the presence of this type of antagonist shows reduced efficacy (= reduced maximal response of agonist), as well as right shift (reduced potency).

3. **Noncompetitive (allosteric) antagonism** (Fig. 5.7): There is flattening of log DRC.

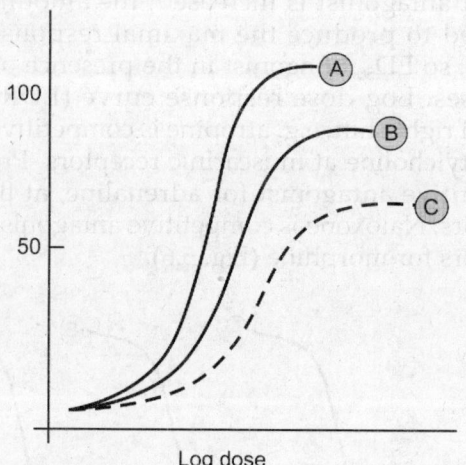

Fig. 5.7: Irreversible/noncompetitive antagonism

A. LDR curve for agonist alone.
B. LDR curve for agonist in presence of irreversible antagonist.
C. LDR curve for agonist plus increasing conc. of irreversible antagonist.

Evaluation of Drug Safety (Fig. 5.8a, b)

$$\text{Therapeutic index (TI)} = \frac{\text{LD}_{50} \text{ (median lethal dose)}}{\text{ED}_{50} \text{ (median effective dose)}}$$

For a safe drug, TI should be at least more than one and hence a drug with larger value of LD_{50} but a smaller value of ED_{50} is considered more safe.

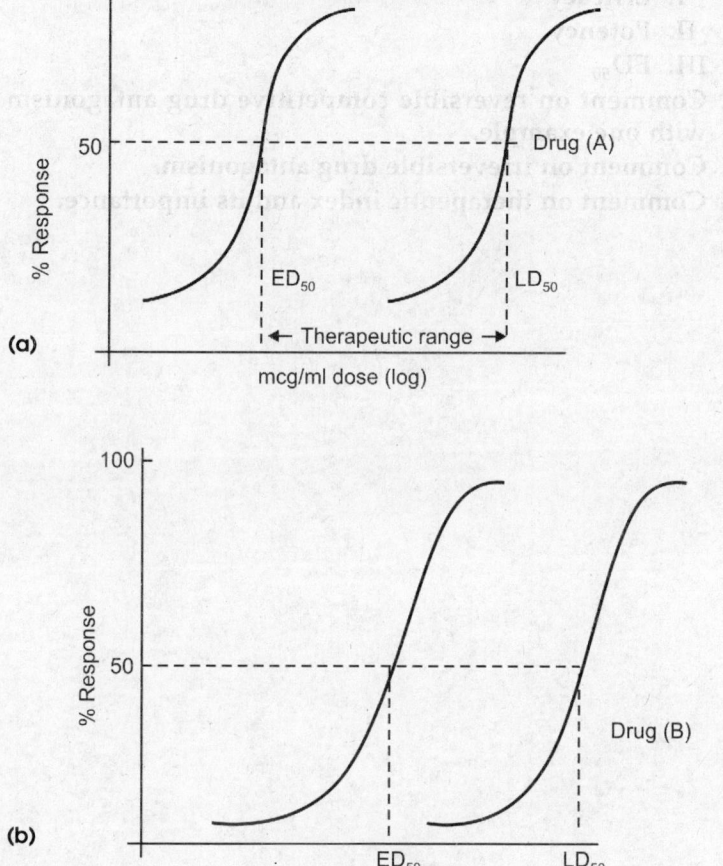

Fig. 5.8: (a) Log DRC of therapeutic and lethal doses of drug (A), **(b)** Log DRC of therapeutic and lethal doses of drug (B)

QUESTIONS

Q 1. What is the difference between graded and quantal DRC?

Q 2. What information could be derived from a log DRC?

Q 3. Define the following:
 I. Efficacy
 II. Potency
 III. ED_{50}

Q 4. Comment on reversible competitive drug antagonism with one example.

Q 5. Comment on irreversible drug antagonism.

Q 6. Comment on therapeutic index and its importance.

Bioassay

ASSAY

Assay is a quantitative estimation of potency of an active substance in unit quantity of preparation.

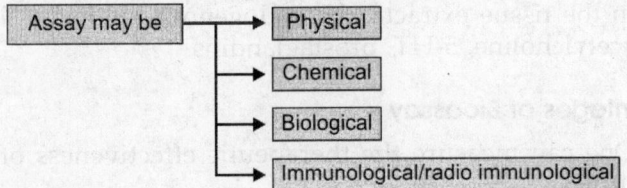

Physical Assay

In physical assay volumetric and gravimetric methods are used to measure potency.

Chemical Assay

Various chemical methods are used to estimate potency of active substance. Most commonly used methods in chemical assay are spectrophotometer or high performance liquid chromatography (HPLC), gas chromatography.

Biological Assay

It means estimation of concentration or potency present in unit quantity of tested substance by measurement of response that it produces on living matter.

Definition of Bioassay

"Bioassay is defined as a comparative assessment of relative potency of a test compound (T) to a standard compound (S) on any living animal or biological tissue."

Indications of Bioassay

1. If the composition or structure of a substance is not known.
2. The chemical structure is known but no simple and specific test is available to assay the drug.
3. The chemical method is too complex and insensitive.
4. The active substance or unknown drug is present in extremely low concentration which cannot be detected by physical and chemical methods.
5. If the active substance can undergo decomposition during isolation or undergo chemical changes by interacting with other chemicals.
6. To estimate the concentration of active substance present in the tissue extracts, the endogenous mediators like—acetylcholine, 5-HT, prostaglandins.

Advantages of Bioassay

1. One can measure the therapeutic effectiveness of new drug.
2. One can measure biological or pharmacological activity of new drug or chemically unidentified compound.
3. Toxicity of new drug can be measured.

Principles of Bioassay

1. Biological activity of unknown drug should always be compared with internationally accepted standard.
2. Species with maximum sensitivity should be used.
3. Bioassay should be designed properly in order to estimate error limit.
4. The method should be reliable, sensitive and reproducible.
5. The biological activity shown by test compound in the living system should closely resemble therapeutic activity of drug.

6. The reference standard in test sample should have similar pharmacological effect and same mode of action so that log DRC (dose response curve) run parallel and their potency ratio can be conventionally compared.

Bioassay is also essential in the development of new drugs. In the preclinical assessment of a new compound, the biological activity is compared with that of known (standard) compound(s), using appropriate test systems. In such studies the test must be simple reproducible and economical.

Types of Bioassay

1. **Quantal (= all or none) bioassay:** The response is either achieved or not achieved, like digitalis produces cardiac arrest in guinea pigs or insulin-induced hypoglycaemic convulsive reaction.

2. **Graded response bioassay:** There is proportionate increase in observed response with a subsequent increase in concentration/dose of drug.

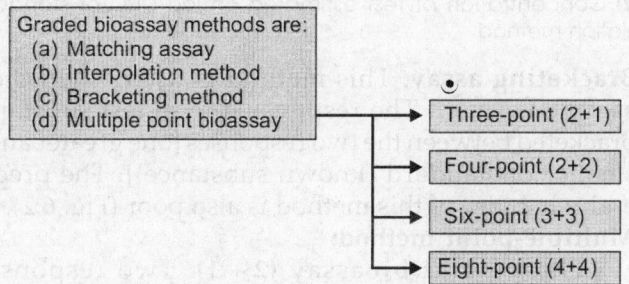

a. **Matching assay:** Used when the test sample is too small. It is most simple type of bioassay. In this type of bioassay, the response of test substance is taken first and the observed response is tried to match with the response of standard drug. Several responses of standard (= known) drug are recorded till a close matching response to that of test substance is observed. A corresponding concentration is thus calculated. Since matching assay does not involve the recording of dose response curve (DRC), the sensitivity of the preparation is not taken into consideration, therefore, the precision and reliability are not very good by this method.

b. **Graphical/interpolation method:** In this type of bioassay, a log dose response curve of standard (known) is first established. Then record 2–3 responses due to test (unknown) substance. The dose of test drug–test response relationship is interpolated from the dose response plot (Fig. 6.1).

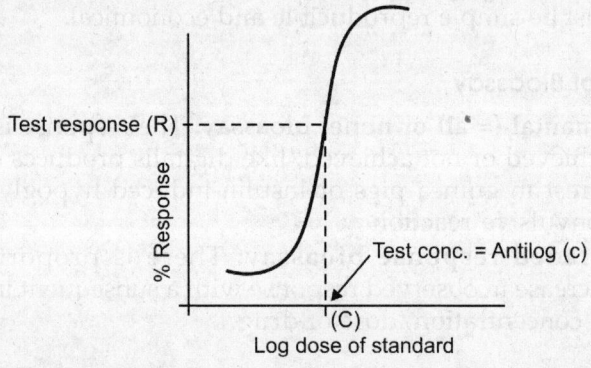

Fig. 6.1: Concentration of test estimated on log DRC of standard by interpolation method

c. **Bracketing assay:** This method is used when the test sample is small. The response due to test substance is bracketed between the two responses [one greater and one smaller of standard (known substance)]. The precision and reliability of this method is also poor (Fig. 6.2).

d. **Multiple-point method:**

   i. **Three-point bioassay (2 + 1):** Two responses of standard (S) and one response of test (T) sample are taken into consideration and test response should be intermediate between the two standard responses.

   ii. **Four-point (2 + 2) bioassay:** Two responses of standard drug and two responses of test substance are used. The selection of two responses of the standard should be such that they are on the linear portion of DRC and also the ratio between the doses should be preferably 1:2. The selection of the test response is determined by hit and trial method so that the responses fall on the linear portion of DRC.

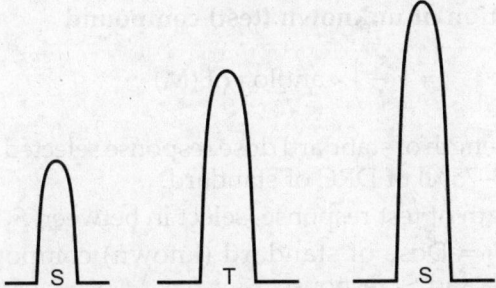

Fig. 6.2: Bracketing method: Test response is bracketed between the smaller and larger response of standard

iii. **Six-point (3 + 3) bioassay:** Three responses of standard and three of test substance are taken. But they are time-consuming processes.

Tissues for Bioassay

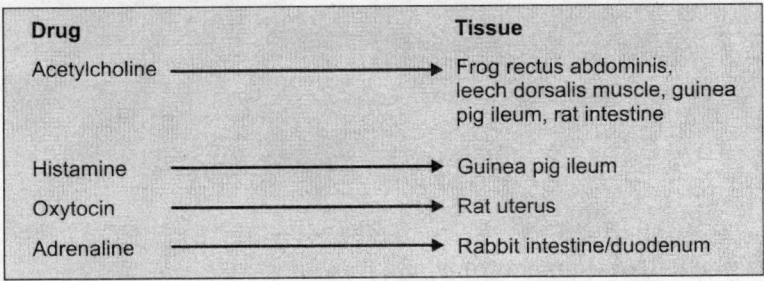

Drug	Tissue
Acetylcholine	Frog rectus abdominis, leech dorsalis muscle, guinea pig ileum, rat intestine
Histamine	Guinea pig ileum
Oxytocin	Rat uterus
Adrenaline	Rabbit intestine/duodenum

Three-point Bioassay

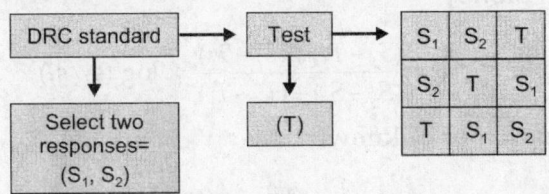

= S_1, S_2, T, S_2, T, S_1, T, S_1, S_2
Then calculate mean of S_1, S_2 and T

Calculation for 3-point assay →

Relative potency (M) = $\dfrac{(T-S_1)}{(S_2-S_1)} \times \log(s_2/s_1)$

Concentration of unknown (test) compound

$$= \left(\frac{s_1}{t}\right) \times \text{antilog of (M)}$$

S_1, S_2 = Length of standard dose response selected from linear portion (25–75%) of DRC of standard.

T = Length of test response, select in between S_1 and S_2.

s_1 and s_2 = Dose of standard (known) compound which produces S_1 and S_2 response.

t = Dose of test (unknown) which produces T response.

Four-point Bioassay

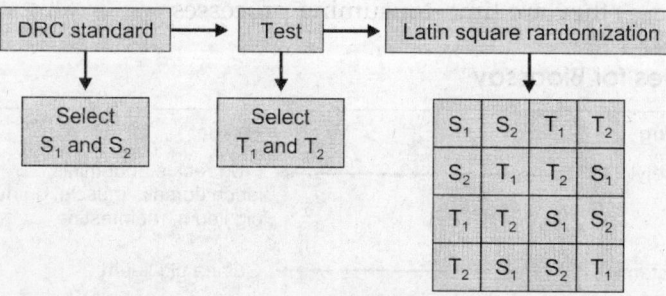

$$= S_1, S_2, T_1, T_2, S_2, T_1, T_2, S_1, T_1, T_2, S_1, S_2, T_2, S_1, S_2, T_1$$

Then calculate mean of S_1, S_2, T_1 and T_2

Relative Potency

$$M = \frac{(S_2 - T_2) + (S_1 - T_1)}{(S_2 - S_1) + (T_2 - T_1)} \times \log(s_2/s_1)$$

Concentration of unknown

$$= \left(\frac{s_1}{t_1}\right) \times \text{antilog of (M)}$$

S_1, S_2 = Length of standard dose response selected from the linear portion of DRC of standard

T_1, T_2 = Length of test dose response selected

s_1, s_2 = Doses of standard, which produced S_1 and S_2 responses

t_1, t_2 = Doses of test, which produced T_1 and T_2 responses

Dose Response Curve (Figs 6.3 and 6.4)

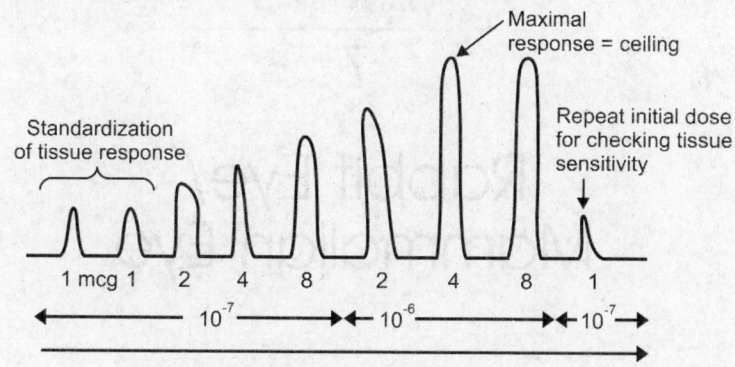

Fig. 6.3: Ascending dose response plot

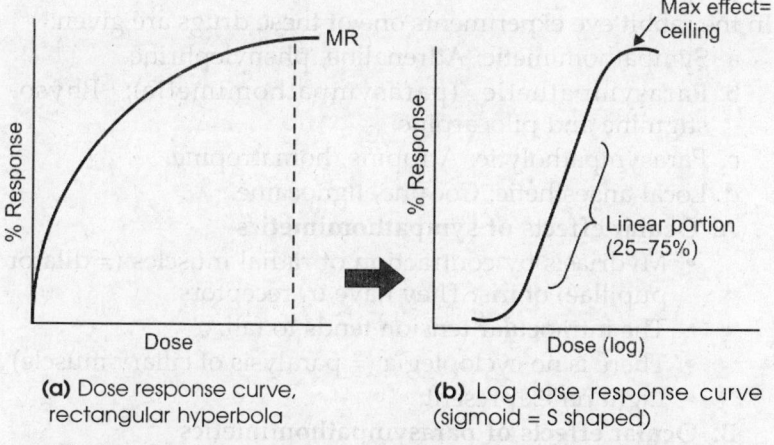

(a) Dose response curve, rectangular hyperbola

(b) Log dose response curve (sigmoid = S shaped)

Fig. 6.4: (a) Dose response curve, **(b)** Log dose response curve

QUESTIONS

Q 1. **Define bioassay. What are the types of bioassay?**
Q 2. **What is the difference between matching assay and bracketing assay?**
Q 3. **What is the difference between matching assay and three-point assay?**
Q 4. **What are the advantages and disadvantages of four-point assay?**

Chapter

7

Rabbit Eye/ Mammalian Eye

In the rabbit eye experiments one of these drugs are given:
 a. Sympathomimetic: Adrenaline, phenylephrine.
 b. Parasympathetic (parasympathomimetic): Physostigmine and pilocarpine
 c. Parasympatholytic: Atropine, homatropine.
 d. Local anaesthetic: Cocaine, lignocaine.

A. Ocular effects of sympathomimetics
 - Mydriasis by contraction of radial muscles (= dilator pupillae) of iris. They have α_1 receptors.
 - The intraocular tension tends to fall.
 - There is no cycloplegia (= paralysis of ciliary muscle)
 - Light reflex present.

B. Ocular effects of parasympathomimetics
 - Miosis due to contraction of circular muscles (sphincter pupillae) of iris.
 - Circular muscle of iris, ciliary muscle and lacrimal gland possess M_3 (muscarinic) receptors.
 - These drugs (parasympathomimetics) cause contraction of circular muscles of iris and ciliary muscle.
 - Contraction of circular muscle of iris causes miosis while contraction of ciliary muscle makes the suspensory ligament of lens loose. This makes the lens more convex and thus the eye is accommodated for near vision (= spasm of accommodation).

- The ciliary muscle contraction also opens the pores of canal of Schlemm which facilitate drainage of aqueous humour leading to reduction of intraocular pressure. (More particularly in the patients suffering from glaucoma.)
- Stimulation of M_3 receptors at lacrimal gland produces lacrimation (due to vasodilation).

C. **Ocular effects of parasympatholytics:** Atropine is the prototype of this group. It antagonises all the actions of parasympathetic muscarinic system. Thus in the eye it causes

- Mydriasis and increases intraocular tension
- Abolition of light reflex
- Cycloplegia: This causes photophobia and blurring of near vision.
- Paralysis of accommodation: Can be anticholinergic side effect of some medications (e.g. antipsychotics, antidepressants).

D. **Ocular effects of local anaesthetics:** Cocaine is a local anaesthetic which is used for ocular anaesthesia. Due to its local anaesthetic property it causes abolition of corneal reflex.

Another important property of cocaine is that it inhibits the reuptake of adrenaline and noradrenaline into peripheral nerve endings. Reuptake is the principal mechanism by which the actions of adrenaline and noradrenaline is terminated. Thus by inhibiting reuptake, cocaine causes sympathomimetic effect like—local vasoconstriction, tachycardia, ↑ BP and mydriasis. Light reflex present.

In the rabbit eye experiments, 4 parameters are studied:

1. Pupil size
2. Light reflex
3. Corneal reflex
4. State of conjunctival vessels.

A. Pupil size: Pupil size is controlled by two groups of muscles of iris (Fig. 7.1)

- 1. Radial muscle (= dilator pupillae) supplied by sympathetic nervous system (cervical sympathetic).
- 2. Circular muscle (= sphincter pupillae) supplied by parasympathetic nervous system (oculomotor).
- Radial muscles have α_1 (adrenergic) receptors.
- Circular muscles have M_3 (muscarinic) receptors.
- Contraction of radial muscles leads to dilation of pupil (= mydriasis), whereas contraction of circular muscles leads to constriction of pupil (miosis).

Active and Passive Miosis

1. Active miosis: Constriction of pupil caused by contraction of sphincter pupillae (= circular muscle) is known as active miosis. It is caused by parasympathomimetic drug, e.g. pilocarpine, physostigmine (= eserine).

2. Passive miosis: Constriction of pupil caused by blockade of action of dilator pupillae (= radial muscles), and unopposed action of sphincter pupillae is known as passive miosis. It is caused by sympatholytic drug, e.g. α-blocker.

Active and Passive Mydriasis

1. Active mydriasis: Dilation of pupil caused by contraction of dilator pupillae is known as active mydriasis and it is caused by sympathomimetic drug like adrenaline, phenylephrine.

2. Passive mydriasis: Caused by blockade of sphincter pupillae by antimuscarinic drug—atropine, and subsequent dilation of pupil due to unopposed action of dilator pupillae.

B. Light reflex: When light is shone in one eye, both the pupils constrict. Constriction of the pupil to which light is shone is known as direct light reflex and that of other pupil is known as consensual (= indirect) light reflex (Fig. 7.2).

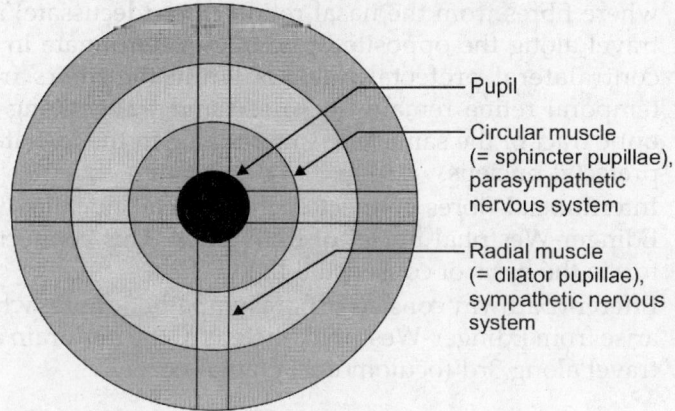

Fig. 7.1: Control of pupil size by iris muscles

Pathway of Light Reflex (Fig. 7.2)

- Light reflex is initiated by rods and cones.
- Afferent fibres extend from retina to pretectal nucleus in midbrain. They travel along optic nerve to optic chiasm

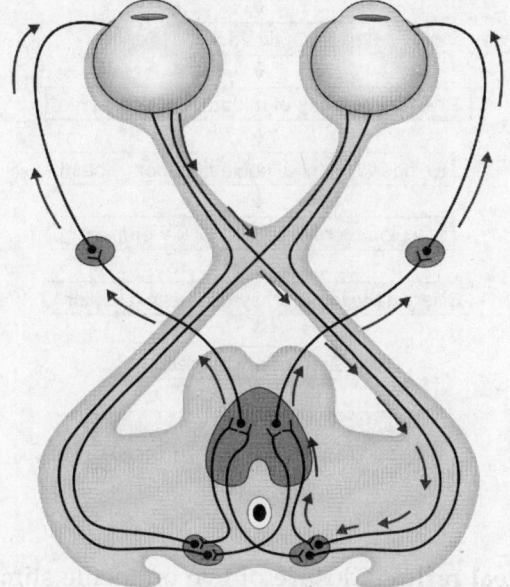

Fig. 7.2: Pathway of light reflex

where fibres from the nasal retina cross (decussate) and travel along the opposite optic tract to terminate in the contralateral pretectal nucleus while the fibers from temporal retina remain uncrossed and travel along the optic tract of the same side to terminate in the ipsilateral pretectal nucleus.

- Internuncial fibres connect each pretectal nucleus with Edinger-Westphal nuclei of both sides. This connection forms the basis of consensual light reflex.
- Efferent pathway consists of parasympathetic fibres which arise from Edinger-Westphal nucleus in the midbrain and travel along 3rd (oculomotor) cranial nerve.

Pathway

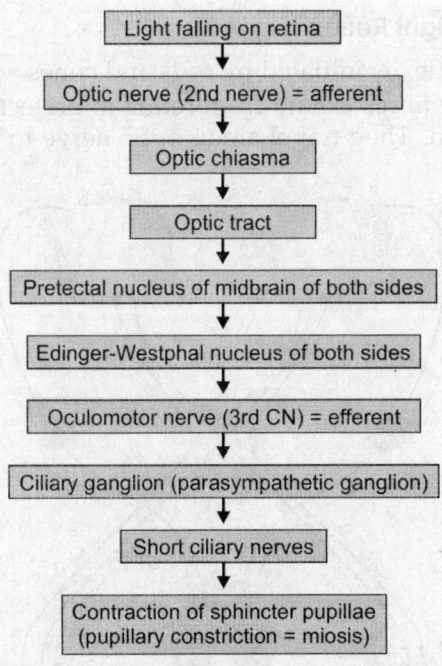

C. Corneal reflex: Closure of eye on tactile stimulation of cornea is corneal reflex.

Pathway

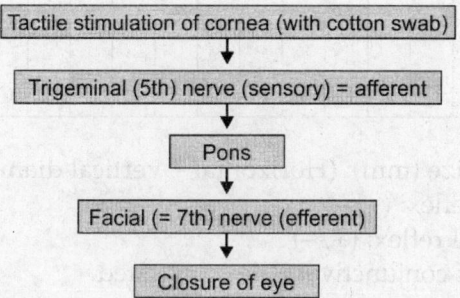

Tactile stimulation of cornea (with cotton swab)
↓
Trigeminal (5th) nerve (sensory) = afferent
↓
Pons
↓
Facial (= 7th) nerve (efferent)
↓
Closure of eye

D. State of conjunctival vessels: Conjunctiva is the outermost layer of eyeball. It covers the sclera. The dilatations of the conjunctival vessels lead to congestion which gives the lower fornix a reddish appearance. The constriction of vessels results in a pale appearance.

Sympathomimetic and parasympatholytic drugs lead to constriction of vessels, whereas parasympathomimetic drug leads to dilatation of vessels.

Experiment no. 1

Object: To study effect of given drugs (miotics, mydriatics and local anaesthetics) on rabbit eye.

Animal: Rabbits.

Requirement: Drugs like physostigmine (1%), pilocarpine (4%), atropine (1%), cocaine (1%) and adrenaline (1%).

Procedure:

- Rabbit is placed on the table and its eyelashes are cut with scissors, one eye is used as test eye (drug) and other eye is used as control eye (distilled water/saline).
- Instill 1–2 drops of drug or saline in the respective eyes.
- Measure the parameters to be observed.

Observations: Four parameters and measured before and every 5 min after instillation for 30 min.

Time (min.)	0		5		10		15		20		25		30	
•Eye C = control, T = test	C	T	C	T	C	T	C	T	C	T	C	T	C	T

1. Pupil size (mm): (Horizontal + vertical diameter)/2
2. Light reflex: (+/−)
3. Corneal reflex: (+/−)
4. State of conjunctiva: Pale/congested.

	Ocular effects of miotics, mydriatics and local anaesthetics				
S. No.	Drug	Pupil size	Light reflex (LR)	Corneal reflex (CR)	State of conjunctival vessels
1.	Pilocarpine	↓ (= miosis)	+	+	Congested
2.	Physostigmine	↓ (= miosis)	+	+	Congested
3.	Phenylephrine or adrenaline	↑ (= mydriasis)	+	+	Pale
4.	Atropine	↑ (= mydriasis)	−	+	Pale
5.	Cocaine	↑ (= mydriasis)	+	−	Pale

(+) = Present
(+) = Abolished
(↑) = Increases
(↓) = Decreases

Results and Conclusion

Clinical Importance

- Miotics are employed in ophthalmological practice to constrict the pupil and to lower intraocular tension in various forms of glaucoma (e.g. physostigmine, pilocarpine).

- Atropine, homatropine and related drugs are used to produce cycloplegia, prior to refraction. They may also be used as mydriatic to permit more complete examination of fundus and to give rest to an inflamed eye. These drugs raise intraocular tension and may precipitate an attack of glaucoma, and therefore, should be used with caution in elderly patients. In such cases it is preferable to use sympathomimetic agents since they have favourable effect on intraocular tension, and also their mydriatic effect is brief and accommodation remain unaffected (e.g. phenylephrine).
- Timolol (β adrenergic antagonist) is employed topically in glaucoma. It reduces production of aqueous humour and does not affect pupillary aperture.

Miotics

1. In glaucoma—miotics increase the tone of ciliary muscle and sphincter pupillae → improved alignment of trabeculae → outflow is increased → IOT (intraocular tension) falls in open angle glaucoma. In primary angle-closure glaucoma, miotics reduce IOT because of their miotic effect by opening the angle of anterior chamber. The mechanical contraction of pupil moves the iris away from the trabecular meshwork.
2. To reverse the effect of mydriatics after refraction testing.
3. To prevent formation of adhesions (= synechiae) between iris-lens and iris-cornea and even to break those which have formed due to iritis, corneal ulcer, etc. A miotic is alternated with a mydriatic.

Mydriatics

1. Tropicamide has the quickest (20–40 min) and briefest (3–6 hours) action; but unreliable cycloplegic. However, it is satisfactory for refraction testing in adults and as a short acting mydriatic for fundoscopy.
2. Other mydriatics → Homatropine, cyclopentolate.
3. For testing error of refraction, both mydriasis and cycloplegia are needed **(diagnostic use)**. Tropicamide having briefer for action has now largely replaced

homatropine for this purpose. These drugs do not cause sufficient cycloplegia in children, so more potent agent like atropine has to be used. [Atropine ointment (1%) applied 24 hours and 2 hours before is often preferred in children below 5 years.]

Therapeutic use: Atropine, because of its long-lasting mydriatic—cycloplegic and local anodyne action on cornea, used in treatment of iritis, iridocyclitis, choroiditis, keratitis, corneal ulcer. It gives rest to intraocular muscles.

Atropinic drugs alternated with a miotic prevent adhesions between iris-lens or iris-cornea and may even break already formed adhesions (= synechiae).

Phenylephrine: Selective α_1 agonist, negligible β action.

Topically used as a nasal decongestant and for producing mydriasis when cycloplegia is not required.

Causes of Pinpoint Pupil

1. Poisoning:
   - Morphine (constricts the pupil by stimulating Edinger-Westphal nucleus).
   - Organophosphate compounds (occasionally unequal).
   - Barbiturates.
   - Carbolic acid (= phenol).
   - Alcohol (late stage of poisoning).
2. Iatrogenic: Overdose of neostigmine in treating myasthenia gravis.
3. Hyperpyrexia: Sunstroke.
4. Pontine haemorrhage (= a type of cerebrovascular accident)
5. Miscellaneous
   - Syringomyelia (a chronic progressive disease of spinal cord characterised by development of cavities = cavitary expansion of cervical cord. There is Horner syndrome in some cases (= miosis, anhidrosis). There is dissociated sensory loss (= loss of pain and temperature with sparing of touch and vibration).
   - Iridocyclitis (narrow, irregular, nonreacting pupil).

Causes of Dilated Pupils

1. Drugs:
   - Belladonna/dhatura
   - Adrenaline/sympathomimetics
   - Atropine/parasympatholytics
   - Cocaine.
2. Sympathetic stimulation
3. Epilepsy
4. Anaemia
5. Optic atrophy
6. Acute congestive glaucoma (vertically oval large immobile pupil)

Hippus

Alternate rhythmic dilation and constriction of pupils.

Causes of Hippus

a. Recovery from 3rd nerve paralysis
b. Syphilis
c. Multiple sclerosis
d. Neoplasms.

Argyll Robertson Pupil

Irregular, unequal, miotic, light reflex absent but accommodation reflex present, poor response to pain and mydriatics.

Causes

1. Neurosyphilis (most common)
2. Encephalitis
3. Chronic alcoholism
4. Diabetes
5. Tumor in brain.
6. Herpes zoster ophthalmicus

Adie's Tonic Pupil

This is a widely dilated circular pupil that reacts very slowly to bright light, but reacts more definitely to accommodation.

Horner's Syndrome

Horner's syndrome occurs due to paralysis of sympathetic fibres resulting in (ptosis, miosis, anhydrosis, enophthalmos and absent ciliospinal reflex).

Ptosis = Drooping of upper eyelid

Miosis = Constriction of pupils.

Anhydrosis = Diminished or complete absence of secretion of sweat.

Enophthalmos = Recession of eyeball into orbit (= opposite to exophthalmos).

Ciliospinal reflex = Dilatation of pupil following stimulation of skin of the neck by pinching or scratching.

QUESTIONS

Q 1. Compare and contrast—active and passive miosis.

Q 2. Compare and contrast—active and passive mydriasis.

Q 3. What do you understand by cycloplegia? Name a mydriatic that is cycloplegic.

Q 4. Name a mydriatic without cycloplegic effect.

Q 5. Comment about the ocular effects of atropine.

Q 6. Comment about the uses of miotics and mydriatics.

Q 7. Draw a flow chart/diagram of visual pathway and light reflex.

Q 8. Draw a flow chart/diagram of pathway of corneal reflex.

Q 9. Enumerate the drugs causing miosis and mydriasis.

Q 10. Make a comparative observation table of miotic, mydriatic and local anaesthetic drug on the four parameters of rabbit eye experiment.

Q 11. What do you understand by glaucoma? Enumerate the drugs used in medical treatment of glaucoma along with their mechanism of actions.

8

Effect of Drugs on Rabbit Ileum by Magnus Method

OBJECT OF EXPERIMENT

To study the effect of spasmogenics and spasmolytics on isolated rabbit ileum preparation.

Apparatus

Dale's organ bath, tuberculin syringe, thermometer, stopwatch, dissecting instruments, etc.

- Animal used—rabbits
- PSS—Tyrode's solution

Drugs

1. Acetylcholine, 50 µg (0.5 ml of 0.01% solution)
2. $BaCl_2$, 5 mg (0.5 ml of 1% solution)
3. Adrenaline, 1 µg (0.1 ml of 1:100,000 solution)
4. Atropine, 250 µg (0.5 ml of 0.01% solution)
5. Papaverine, 500 µg (0.5 ml of 1:1000 solution)

   µg = microgram (mcg)

Parameters to be Studied

1. Tone—partial state of contraction of a tissue at rest (indicated by baseline of a contraction tracing).
2. Amplitude—height of contraction.
3. Rate—number of contraction in unit time. It is shown by the distance between contractions.

Procedure

A piece of ileum (2–3 cm) is provided from a freshly sacrificed rabbit by injecting a large dose of anaesthetic, which has been fasted for 24 hours. The piece of ileum is suspended in the inner bath filled with PSS (Tyrode's solution) at 36–37°C. One end of the ileum is tied to the bent aeration tube and the other end is attached with frontal writing lever by means of a thread. The lever must be balanced with plasticine or moulding clay with a proper magnification of the lever (5–7 times), so that only slight increase in tension in the gut is required to move it. The speed of the drum is kept slow. Keep the outer bath temperature to 37–38°C and ensure continuous slow air supply to the suspended tissue. The drugs are added only after the preparation has stabilized. Always take a control tracing before adding the drug. Drugs should be washed out at least three to four times once a suitable record is obtained.

Two types of muscles are found in GIT:
a. Circular
b. Longitudinal

Four types of movements in GIT:
a. Pendular (produced by longitudinal muscle, mix food).
b. Segmental (produced due to circular muscle contraction).
c. Peristalsis (help in mixing and propagation of food).
d. Antiperistalsis (help in mixing and propagation of food).

- Two types of drugs acting on intestine are studied. **(GIT muscles are smooth muscles)**
  1. **Spasmogenic drugs:** ↑tone and ↑ amplitude of GIT contractions, ↑ spasm of GIT, e.g.
     a. ACh (indirectly acting via receptor)
     b. Directly acting drugs $BaCl_2$.
  2. **Spasmolytic drugs:** ↓spasm of intestine by decreasing tone and amplitude.
     a. Indirectly acting = Adrenaline (α, β agonist), atropine (muscarinic antagonist).
     b. Directly acting = Papaverine, nitrates.

Clinical Importance
1. Spasmogenic drugs used in paralytic ileus.
2. Spasmolytic drugs used in colics.

Precautions During Experiment

1. Tissue should be held gently, not to be overstretched.
2. Constant aeration throughout experiment (for mixing of drug properly)
3. Temperature of bath (maintained at 37°–38°C)
4. Not to change the speed of drum (make it constant = slow).
5. Next drug to be added when control tracing is recorded.

S. No.	Drug	Tone	Ampl.	Result
1.	ACh	↑	↑	Spasmogenic
2.	BaCl$_2$	↑	↑	Spasmogenic
3.	Adrenaline	↓	↓	Spasmolytic
4.	Atropine	↓	↓	Spasmolytic
5.	Papaverine	↓	↓	Spasmolytic

Object

To demonstrate the action of unknown drugs on the isolated gut. Determine its nature and probable site of action.

Step I: Nature of action: Add 0.5 ml of unknown drug. Determine whether it stimulates or depresses the movements of gut. If no clear-cut effect is observed, then repeat the dose.

Step II: Site of action:
  A. **If the unknown drug is stimulant, there are 2 possibilities**
   i. Indirectly acting (acting on receptors), parasympathomimetics, e.g. ACh, carbachol.
   ii. Directly acting stimulant drug for musculature BaCl$_2$.
      → **To establish the site of action of the drug**
      1. **Observe the type of tracing:** ACh, which acts on cholinergic receptors, has a short duration of action,

while directly acting drug produces long-lasting spasmodic contraction.

2. **Add 0.5 ml of atropine to the same inner bath:** Abolition of the stimulation suggests that the unknown drug was parasympathomimetic. This is confirmed by a second addition of 0.5 ml of unknown drug. After atropine, a parasympatho-mimetic drug will not produce stimulation. The directly acting drugs ($BaCl_2$) produce stimulation, even after atropine.

B. **If the unknown drug produces depression, possibilities are:**
   i. **Indirectly acting drug (acting on receptors)**
      • Sympathomimetic = Adrenaline
      • Parasympatholytic = Atropine
   ii. **Directly acting drug (acting on musculature)—** Papaverine.   ●

To establish site of action of unknown drug

1. **Observe the type of tracing:** The depression produced by adrenaline is short lived. Atropine abolishes only the abnormal movements of gut. The directly acting papaverine produces a long-lasting depression.

2. After observing the effect of unknown drug, add 0.5 ml acetylcholine to the same bath. If stimulation occurs, the unknown drug may be adrenaline. If on adding of 0.5 ml acetylcholine, there is no change of effect, it may be atropine or papaverine. Now add 0.5 ml $BaCl_2$, which will stimulate if the unknown drug is atropine. If $BaCl_2$ fails to stimulate, the unknown drug is papaverine.

Step III: Direct matching with known sample.

Experiment No. 1

To study the action of known drugs (spasmogenics) on the motility of isolated rabbit gut preparation.

Prepare the experiment as described. Add the drugs in the following order:

a. Acetylcholine (0.1%)—0.5 ml. Repeat the dose if necessary.

b. Atropine (0.5%)—0.5 ml. It is added to block the muscarinic receptors.
c. Acetylcholine (0.1%)—0.5 ml is again added in inner bath, without washing after atropine addition.
d. Barium chloride (1%)—0.5 ml.

Experiment No. 2

To study the action of known drugs (spasmolytics) on the motility of isolated rabbit gut preparation.

Prepare the experiment as described. Add the drugs in the following order:

a. Adrenaline (1:100000)—0.5 ml. Repeat the dose—if necessary.
b. Atropine (0.5%)—0.5 ml.
c. Papaverine (1: 1000)—0.5 ml.

Experiment No. 3

To study the action of unknown drugs (spasmogenic or spasmolytic) on the motility of isolated rabbit gut preparation.

Prepare the experiment as described.

QUESTIONS

Q 1. Name the types of GIT movements.
Q 2. Which part of GIT is selected for rabbit gut experiment and why?
Q 3. Name the lever, its magnification, and PSS used in this experiment.
Q 4. Why we maintain the temperature of organ bath throughout this experiment?
Q 5. Name some spasmogenic and spasmolytic drugs.
Q 6. How will you differentiate the nature and site of action of spasmogenic drugs in rabbit gut experiments?
Q 7. How will you differentiate the nature and site of action of spasmolytic drugs in rabbit gut experiments?
Q 8. Write the composition of Tyrode solution.

9

Study of Autonomic Drugs on Perfused Frog Heart

Procedure: Pith the brain and spinal cord of a frog (double pithing) and pin it on the board in supine position. Remove the abdominal wall by V-shaped incision from the pelvis to pectoral girdle. Expose the heart. Remove pericardium. Insert a small heart hook through ventricular apex and with the ligature attached to it, pull the heart anteriorly. Sinus venosus is cannulated using a glass cannula (= Syme's cannula) and secured with thread. Then the heart is perfused with Ringer solution through sinus venosus. Truncus arteriosus of both sides are cut and a curved needle is inserted in the apex and attached to a heart lever for recording contractions on the smoked paper pasted over the drum of a kymograph. Starling heart lever is used (it records fast contractions). Lever should be horizontal. Normal contractions are recorded followed by effect of drugs.

Important

   a. Frog heart is three-chambered → two atria and one ventricle.
   b. Ventricle contains mix blood.
   c. Superior and inferior vena cava open into sinus venosus. Venous blood flows from sinus venosus to right atrium and from right atrium to ventricle. Arterial blood comes from left atrium into ventricle. Ventricle pumps mixed blood to bulbous aorta. Bulbous aorta have spiral valve

68

that directs arterial blood to body and venous blood to lungs through pulmonary arteries.

Parameters Observed in a Curve/Tracing (Fig. 9.1)

1. **Tone:** Tone is defined as partial state of contraction. It is indicated by baseline of the tracing. Increase of tone as shown by rise of baseline indicates stimulation while decrease as shown by lowering of baseline indicates depression. Sometimes when a drug is given, cardiac arrest occurs, then the stimulant or depressant nature of the drug is decided by rise or fall of the baseline respectively.

2. **Amplitude of contraction:** Indicated by total height of curve. Increase means forceful contraction and stimulation.

3. **Rate:** Increase is shown by contractions growing closer to each other. Decrease is shown by contractions growing far apart.

→ Upward stroke in the tracing indicates systole while downward stroke indicates diastole.

→ **Inject the drugs in the following order:**

1. Adrenaline (0.01%) = 0.25 ml
2. Calcium chloride (1%) = 0.5 ml
3. Propranolol (0.1%) = 0.5 ml

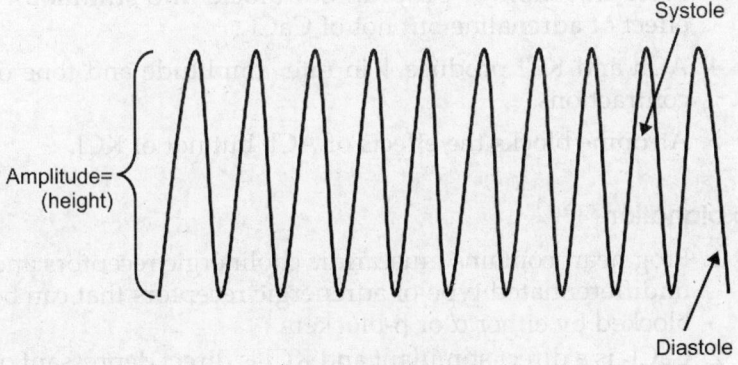

Fig. 9.1: Normal curve

After 2 minutes (without washing)

4. Adrenaline (0.01%) = 0.25 ml
5. Calcium chloride (1%) = 0.5 ml
6. Calcium chloride (1%) = 2 ml

Wash

1. Acetylcholine (0.1%) = 0.25 ml
2. Potassium chloride (2%) = 0.25 ml
3. Atropine (0.5%) = 0.25 ml

After 2 minutes (without washing)

4. Acetylcholine (0.1%) = 0.25 ml
5. Potassium chloride (2%) = 0.5 ml

Observations

1. Injection of adrenaline in perfusate (frog Ringer's solution) increases rate, amplitude and tone of contractions.
2. Injection of $CaCl_2$ increases tone of contraction. The effect on rate and amplitude vary. With low dose increase in rate and amplitude occurs. When the dose is increased, it results in decrease in rate and amplitude. Cardiac arrest occurs when high dose is used.
3. Prior injection of propranolol blocks the stimulatory effect of adrenaline but not of $CaCl_2$.
4. ACh and KCl produce ↓ in rate, amplitude and tone of contractions.
5. Atropine blocks the effects of ACh but not of KCl.

Explanation

1. Frog heart contains muscarinic cholinergic receptors and undifferentiated type of adrenergic receptors that can be blocked by either α or β-blockers.
2. $CaCl_2$ is a direct stimulant and KCl is direct depressant of frog heart muscle contractions.

3.

Rate	↑	↓	↓
Amplitude	↑	↓	↓
Tone	↑	↓	↑
Conclusion	(S)	(D)	(S)

(S) = Stimulant
(D) = Depressant

→ **Thus tone is the most important parameter to determine whether the drug is stimulant or depressant in nature** (Fig. 9.2).

Drug	Amplitude	Tone	Frequency (= rate)
Adrenaline	↑	↑	↑
ACh	↓	↓	↓
CaCl$_2$ (low dose)	↑	↑	↑
CaCl$_2$ (high dose)	↓	↑	↓
KCl	↓	↓	↓

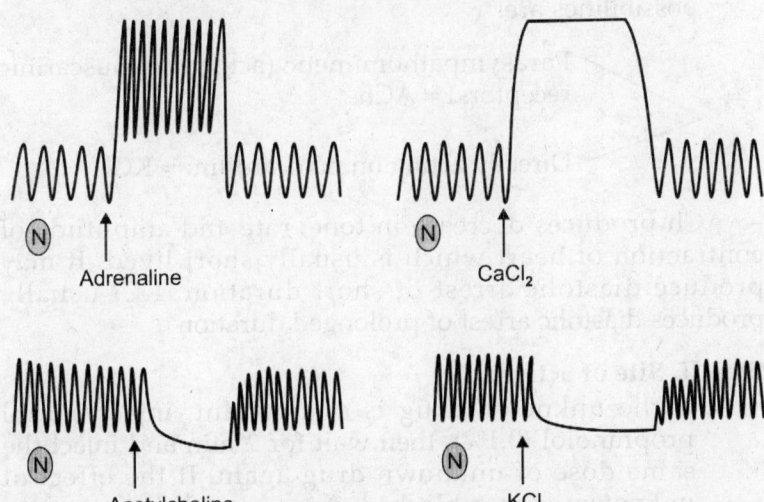

Fig. 9.2: Cardiac stimulants and depressants: Effect on tone, amplitude and rate

Object

To demonstrate the action of unknown drug on frog heart. Determine its nature and probable site of Action (Fig. 9.3).

Step I. Nature of action: Inject 0.25 ml of unknown drug. If there is any effect, repeat the same dose to confirm the effect. If no response, then inject higher dose.

a. If the unknown drug produces a stimulant effect it may be

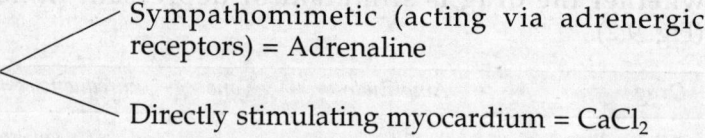

Sympathomimetic (acting via adrenergic receptors) = Adrenaline

Directly stimulating myocardium = $CaCl_2$

→ Adrenaline may not produce much effect on tone of heart, while it produces marked increase rate and amplitude of contraction. $CaCl_2$ produces marked increase in the tone of heart, while rate and amplitude may decrease. It may produce *systolic arrest*.

b. If the unknown drug produces a depressant effect, the possibilities are:

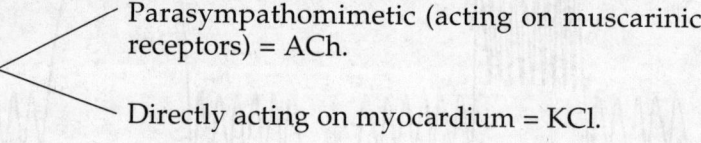

Parasympathomimetic (acting on muscarinic receptors) = ACh.

Directly acting on myocardium = KCl.

→ ACh produces decrease in tone; rate and amplitude of contraction of heart which is usually short lived. It may produce diastolic arrest of short duration. KCl usually produces diastolic arrest of prolonged duration.

Step II. Site of action:

A. If the unknown drug is a stimulant, inject 0.5 ml propranolol (0.1%), then wait for 2 min and inject the same dose of unknown drug again. If the effect of unknown drug is blocked, it is sympathomimetic, i.e. adrenaline. If the stimulant effect of unknown drug is not blocked by propranolol, it is a direct stimulant ($CaCl_2$).

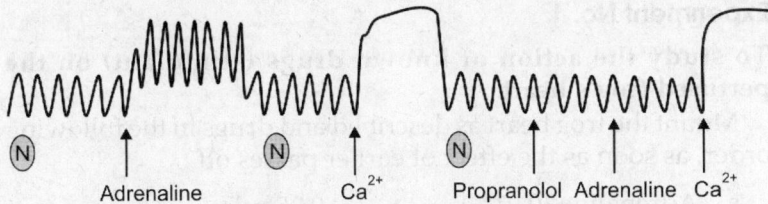

(a) Effect of cardiac stimulants on isolated and perfused frog heart

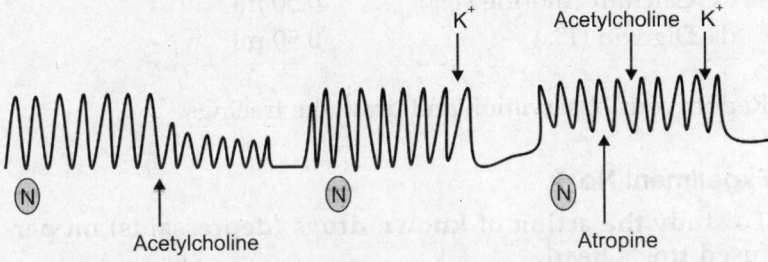

(b) Effect of cardiac depressants on isolated and perfused frog heart

Fig. 9.3

B. If unknown drug is a depressant, inject 0.5 ml of atropine (0.5%), wait for 2 min, and inject the same dose of unknown drug again. If the effect of unknown drug is blocked, it is parasympathomimetic acting through muscarinic cholinergic receptors, i.e. ACh. If the depressant effect of unknown drug is not blocked by atropine, it is a direct acting depressant (KCl).

Step III: Direct matching with known drug. Take a known sample of the probable drug found by you. Inject an equivalent amount and compare the effects with that of unknown drug.

Composition of frog Ringer solution	
Sodium chloride	= 6.5 gm
Potassium chloride	= 0.14 gm
Calcium chloride	= 0.12 gm
Sodium dihydrogen phosphate	= 0.008 gm
Sodium bicarbonate	= 0.2 gm
Glucose	= 2.0 gm
Distilled water	= up to 1000 ml

Experiment No. 1

To study the action of known drugs (stimulant) on the perfused frog's heart.

Mount the frog heart as described and drugs in the following order, as soon as the effect of earlier passes off.

a. Adrenaline (0.01%)   0.25 ml
b. Atropine (0.5%)   0.25 ml
c. Calcium chloride (1%)   0.50 ml
d. Digoxin (1%)   0.50 ml

Report your observation and draw the tracings.

Experiment No. 2

To study the action of known drugs (depressants) on perfused frog's heart.

Prepare the heart as described and inject the drugs in the following orders:

a. Acetylcholine (0.1%)   0.5 ml
b. Potassium chloride (2%)   0.5 ml
c. Atropine (0.5%)   0.5 ml
d. Acetylcholine (0.1%)   0.5 ml
e. Potassium chloride (2%)   0.5 ml

Observe the type of tracing and report your observation.

Experiment No. 3

To study the nature and site of action of unknown drugs (stimulant or depressant) on the perfused frog's heart.

QUESTIONS

Q 1. **Enumerate some cardiac stimulants and depressants.**
Q 2. **Comment on the cardiac actions of cholinomimetics/ acetylcholine.**
Q 3. **Comment on the cardiac actions of atropine.**

Q 4. Comment on the cardiac actions of sympathomimetics/ adrenaline.

Q 5. Comment on the cardiac actions of propranolol.

Q 6. Comment on the cardiac actions of calcium chloride and potassium chloride.

Q 7. Write the composition of frog Ringer solution.

Q 8. Enumerate the cardiovascular uses of atropine and propranolol.

Q 9. How will you differentiate the nature and site of action of cardiac stimulants on perfused frog heart?

Q 10. How will you differentiate the nature and site of action of cardiac depressants on perfused frog heart?

10

Study of Autonomic Drugs on Mammalian Blood Pressure

Object: To study the effect of various drugs on dog blood pressure (BP).

Apparatus: Research kymograph, operation table, U-shaped mercury manometer, tuberculin syringe, burette, arterial, venous and tracheal cannula, connecting rubber tube, dissecting instruments, cotton and thread.

Procedure: A healthy dog is weighed and anaesthetized with pentobarbitone sodium (25 mg/kg IV). After the animal has been anaesthetized, it is mounted on operation table in supine position. Four limbs are tied to four corners of operation table. After that femoral vein is exposed in thigh region and venous cannula is inserted in the vein. Venous cannula is connected to a burette with the help of rubber tubing which contains normal saline. This route is used for injecting drugs IV.

After that a midline incision is given in neck. Skin and fascia reflected, muscles are separated and trachea is exposed. After exposing trachea, search for carotid artery lying in deeper tissue on the side of trachea. An arterial cannula (heparinised) is inserted in the carotid artery and this cannula is connected to a mercury manometer with the help of pressure rubber tubing. This set is used for recording of BP on drum. A partial transverse cut is given in trachea and a Y-shaped tracheal cannula is inserted in the lumen of trachea and connected to a respiratory pump.

→ The drugs are given IV through femoral vein.

Part A

1. Inject rapidly 2 mcg/kg acetylcholine (100 mcg/ml sol.): If this dose does not elicit a fall in BP of at least 30 mmHg in BP, increase the dose of ACh; until it does. This is the standard vasodepressor dose. After then, wait for BP to come to normal.
2. Inject rapidly 0.5 mcg/kg carbachol (20 mcg/ml sol.): If the fall in BP is not equivalent to that caused by standard vasodepressor dose of ACh, increase accordingly. Compare with step 1 and analyse.

Part B

1. Inject 1 mg/kg physostigmine (reversible inhibitor of acetylcholinesterase enzyme).
2. Inject standard vasodepressor dose of ACh and carbachol.
3. Compare and explain the differences observed after physostigmine.
4. Atropinize the dog (1 mg/kg IV) slowly over 5 minutes. Then wait for another 3–5 minutes. Inadequate atropinization is indicated by absence of marked mydriasis and presence of pupillary light reflex to strong light. The dog may require a second dose of atropine (0.5 mg/kg), if there is insufficient atropinization.
5. Inject: (a) The standard vasodepressor dose of ACh.
   Inject: (b) Standard vasodepressor dose of carbachol.
   Inject: (c) Five times the standard vasodepressor dose of ACh and carbachol.

Explain which of the observed effects are Muscarinic and which are Nicotinic in nature.

Part C

1. Inject epinephrine 2 mcg/kg.
2. Inject phenylephine 5 mcg/kg (α_1 agonist)
3. Inject isoprenaline 1 mcg/kg
4. Inject prazosin (α_1 antagonist) 1 mg/kg IV slowly, then wait for 15 min.
5. Repeat epinephrine 2 mcg/kg.
6. Repeat phenylephrine 5 mcg/kg.
7. Repeat isoprenaline 1 mcg/kg.

8. Inject propranolol (1 mg/kg IV slowly) and wait for 10 min.
9. Repeat epinephrine 2 mcg/kg.
10. Repeat isoprenaline 1 mcg/kg.

Explanations

After IV administration of ACh, the BP falls rapidly. This fall is proportional to the dose injected (and if extremely high doses are injected, cardiac arrest in diastole may occur).The actions of carbachol (and other cholinomimetic drugs) is similar on heart and BP. Cholinomimetics reduce HR, force of contraction and CO and also produce vasodilatation due to which BP falls. These events are mediated by vagus nerve in heart and through G-protein/nitric oxide (NO) mechanism in case of blood vessels.

The differences in actions of ACh and carbachol

a. ACh produces a sharp fall in BP, while the fall in BP produced by carbachol is less steep (Fig. 10.1).
b. The duration of action of ACh is smaller as compared to carbachol.

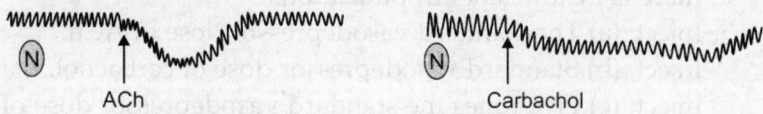

ACh   Carbachol

Fig. 10.1: Effect of cholinomimetics on BP

- Injection of ACh after pretreatment with physostigmine prolongs the duration of effect of ACh by preventing its metabolism by AChE (acetylcholinesterase). The effect of carbachol remains unchanged as it is not metabolized by AChE.
- Atropinization is done to block muscarinic cholinergic receptors. For this purpose atropine is given slow IV over a period of 3–5 min (because quick IV injection of atropine can cause cardiac slowing and even cardiac arrest due to its direct depressant effect on myocardium).
- Injection of 5 times higher dose of ACh in atropinized animals exhibit nicotinic effects of ACh. Excitation of

nicotinic receptors at NM junction (neuromuscular junction) produces muscle twitching. Nicotinic receptors of the ganglia are also excited due to which sympathetic stimulation occurs resulting in rise of BP and HR.

- Injection of epinephrine and norepinephrine produces rise of BP.
- If the vagi are intact, reflex bradycardia is seen during BP elevation produced by norepinephrine. Injection of epinephrine also produces reflex bradycardia that is masked by its direct cardiac stimulant (β_1 effect). In animals having bilateral vagotomy, no reflex bradycardia is seen.
- When epinephrine is injected, a biphasic response can be seen, in which after the initial rise of BP, fall in BP occurs, which is due to vasodilatation produced by β_2 adrenergic receptor stimulation (the effect on α-receptors is short lived while that on β are sustained) (Figs 10.2 and 10.4a).
- Phenylephrine (α_1 agonist) produces effects similar to NE (Fig. 10.3a).
- Isoprenaline, being a β-agonist, produces fall in BP (β_2 effect) and marked tachycardia (β_1 effect) (Fig. 10.3b).
- Injection of muscarinic agonists like acetylcholine and β-agonists like isoprenaline both produce fall in BP. The only difference is that muscarinic agonists (ACh) produce bradycardia, while β-agonists (isoprenaline) produce tachycardia.

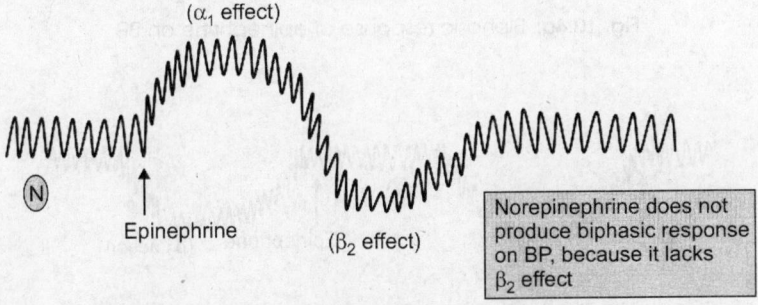

(α_1 effect)

Ⓝ

Epinephrine

(β_2 effect)

Norepinephrine does not produce biphasic response on BP, because it lacks β_2 effect

Fig. 10.2: Epinephrine—biphasic response on BP

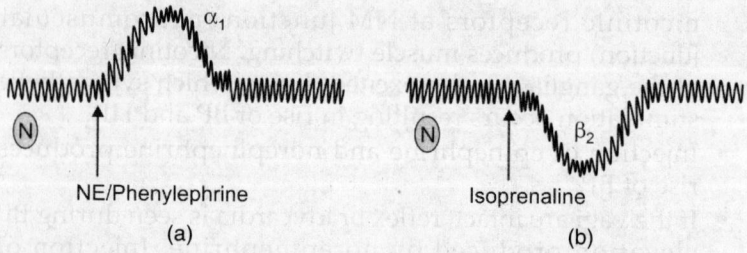

Fig. 10.3: Effect of (a) NE/Phenylephrine and (b) isoprenaline on BP

Prazosin (α_1-antagonist) (Fig. 10.4): It blocks α_1 receptors in vessel walls but has no effect on cardiac β_1 receptors. Due to blockade of α_1 receptors, fall of BP occurs. Phenylephrine and norepinephrine do not produce any effect in such animals because their site of action is already blocked. Epinephrine also fails to produce any rise of BP but the β effect produces both tachycardia (β_1 effect) and fall in BP (β_2 effect). This reversal of epinephrine effect action from rise in BP to fall in BP after administration of α_1-antagonist is known as **Dale's vasomotor reversal phenomenon** (Fig. 10.4b).

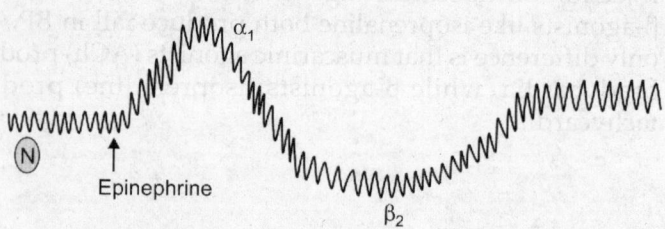

Fig. 10.4a: Biphasic response of epinephrine on BP

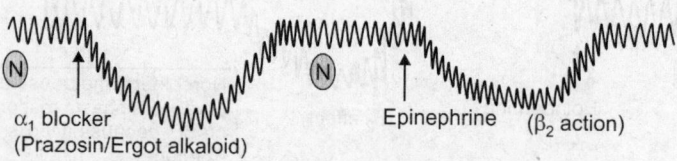

Fig. 10.4b: Dale's vasomotor reversal

The fall in BP produced by isoprenaline (β agonist) remains unchanged in such animals (Fig. 10.5).

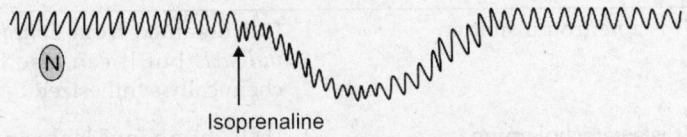

Fig. 10.5: Effect of isoprenaline on BP in the presence of α_1 antagonist

Injection of propranolol produces fall in BP and bradycardia and blocks the fall in BP produced by epinephrine and isoprenaline in these animals (re-reversal) (Fig. 10.6).

After the experiment, animal is euthanised by high dose of anaesthetic.

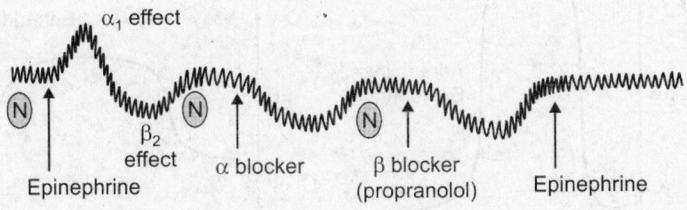

Fig. 10.6a: Re-reversal

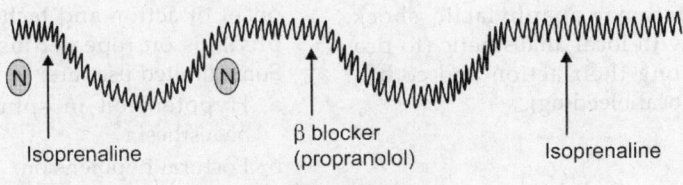

Fig. 10.6b: Re-reversal

Exercise: To differentiate between epinephrine and ephedrine:

Epinephrine	Ephedrine
1. It is a neurotransmitter.	1. It is obtained from *Ephedra vulgaris* but it can also be chemically synthesized
2. It is a catecholamine.	2. It is a phenyl-isopropyl amine.
3. It is directly acting sympatho-mimetic agent (= acts on receptors α_1, α_2, β_1, β_2 and weakly β_3).	3. Mixed action, indirectly by causing release of NE. Directly by acting on adrenoceptors.
4. Rapidly degraded by MAO and COMT, therefore, action is short and the drug is not effective orally.	4. Resistant to MAO, effective orally, prolonged action.

BP — Adrenaline= Epinephrine / Time	BP — Ephedrine / Time

5. More potent.	5. 100 times less potent than epinephrine.
6. Used in cardiac arrest, bronchial asthma, anaphylactic shock, with local anaesthetic (to prolong their action and control local bleeding).	6. Use is limited because slow onset of action and tachyphylaxis on repeated use. Some limited uses are: a. Hypotension in spinal anaesthesia b. Postural hypotension.

Tachyphylaxis (Fig. 10.7)

Tachy – fast, phylaxis = prevention.

Definition: Tachyphylaxis is rapid development of tolerance, when doses of drug are repeated in quick succession. This results in marked reduction in response.

Seen in indirectly acting and mixed acting sympathomimetic drugs.

E.g.

Indirectly acting = tyramine, amphetamine, methamphetamine.

Mixed acting = Ephedrine.

Mechanism: In case of indirectly acting agent, it is due to depletion of NE stores from sympathetic nerve endings. In case of mixed acting agents, it could be due to slow release of transmitter or due to internalization of receptors (= downregulation).

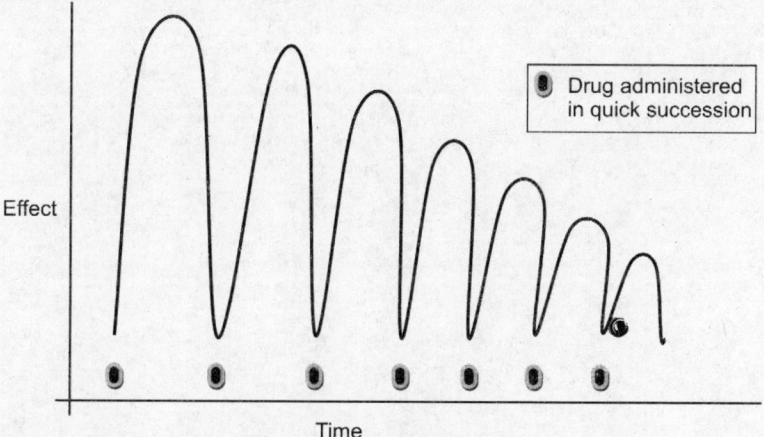

Fig. 10.7: Tachyphylaxis

QUESTIONS

Q 1. What is the effect of cholinomimetics on BP?

Q 2. What is the effect of atropine on BP?

Q 3. What is the effect of adrenaline, noradrenaline and isoprenaline on BP?

Q 4. What is the effect of alpha blockers on BP?

Q 5. What is the effect of beta blockers on BP?

Q 6. Biphasic response on BP is seen with adrenaline and not with noradrenaline, explain.

Q 7. What do you understand by tachyphylaxis? Which drug shows this effect in dog BP experiment? What is the mechanism behind tachyphylaxis?

Q 8. What do you understand by ganglionic action of acetylcholine? Explain it.

Q 9. What do you understand by Dale's vasomotor reversal? Explain it.

11

Frog's Rectus Experiments

METHOD

Pith a frog, lay it dorsally on a frog board. Cut away the abdominal skin and expose the rectus muscle, now dissect the rectus muscle from the pelvis to the pectoral girdle. Bisect it to take out one portion and keep in frog's Ringer solution. A thread is sewn through each end and the muscle is then fixed in the Dale's organ bath by fixing one end to the aeration tube and the other end to the frontal writing lever. Fill the bath with Ringer's solution. For relaxation of the muscle a weight of approximately 0.5 to 1 gm is hanged between fulcrum and writing point for about 30–45 minutes. Magnification is adjusted to about 5–7 times. Ringer's solution changed 2–3 times during relaxation. Now remove the weight and the muscle is ready for experiment. The effect of drug is observed for a period of 90 seconds and then washed, followed by gap of relaxation of 3 minutes each time. Tracings are recorded on a drum.

Experiment 1

To study the effect of graded doses of acetylcholine on isolated frog's rectus muscle preparation.

Prepare the experiment as described. Add 1 µg of acetylcholine to observe the sensitivity of the muscle. A contraction is seen with acetylcholine. Repeat the same dose of acetylcholine to confirm the stability of the preparation.

A similar response shows that the preparation is stable and the effect is reproducible. Acetylcholine is then added in doubling doses to get a log dose response (Sigmoid curve). After a particular dose further addition of acetylcholine did not show increased height of contraction. This is termed maximum response (ceiling response).

Measure the height of contraction of each dose and the dose response curve on a graph.

The effect (contraction) due to acetylcholine is nicotinic N_M receptors on skeletal muscle (rectus).

Experiment 2

To study the effect of unknown drug on acetylcholine-induced contraction on isolated frog's rectus preparation.

Prepare the experiment as described.

Confirm the sensitivity, the stability of the preparation, add graded dose of acetylcholine to show the response.

Now add 0.5 ml of unknown drug and wait for about 5 minutes, repeat the same dose of acetylcholine in graded fashion.

Observe the Tracings

1. Decreased effect of acetylcholine indicates that unknown drug is neuromuscular blocker (skeletal muscle relaxant), e.g. d-tubocurarine, gallamine, pancuronium, etc.
2. Enhanced effect of acetylcholine (potentiation) indicates that the unknown drug is an anticholinesterase, e.g. physostigmine, etc. Plot the dose response of acetylcholine before and after the treatment with unknown drug.

QUESTIONS

Q 1. Temperature maintenance is not necessary in frog rectus abdominis experiments. Why?

Q 2. What is the purpose of aeration in inner organ bath?

Q 3. Which PSS and lever is used in this experiment?

Q 4. What do you understand by potentiation and antagonism?

Q 5. Name the drugs showing potentiation and antagonism
in frog rectus experiment.

Q 6. Name the transmitter and receptor involved in skeletal
muscle contraction at neuromuscular junction.

Q 7. Why we put additional weight of about one gram on
long arm of lever?

Q 8. Name some tissues utilized for *in vitro* study of
acetylcholine.

Q 9. What effects are seen on log DRC in case of potentiation and antagonism?

Q 10. Enumerate the neuromuscular blockers.

12

Evaluation of Local Anaesthetics and Analgesics

LOCAL ANAESTHETICS

These are drugs which are applied topically or injected locally, block nerve conduction and cause reversible loss of all sensations in the parts supplied by nerve.

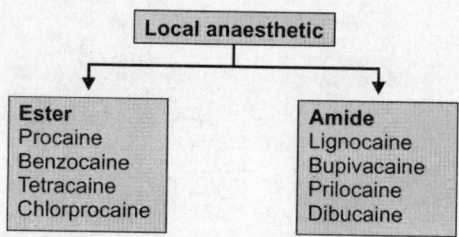

Local anaesthetic	
Ester Procaine Benzocaine Tetracaine Chlorprocaine	**Amide** Lignocaine Bupivacaine Prilocaine Dibucaine

Mechanism of Action

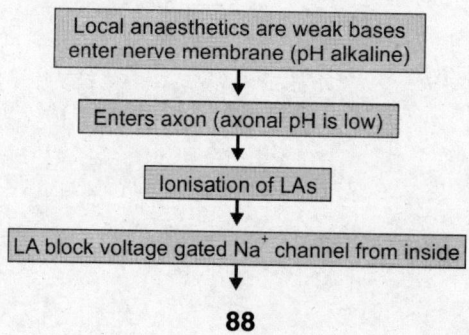

Local anaesthetics are weak bases enter nerve membrane (pH alkaline)

↓

Enters axon (axonal pH is low)

↓

Ionisation of LAs

↓

LA block voltage gated Na^+ channel from inside

↓

88

(Contd.)

(Contd.)

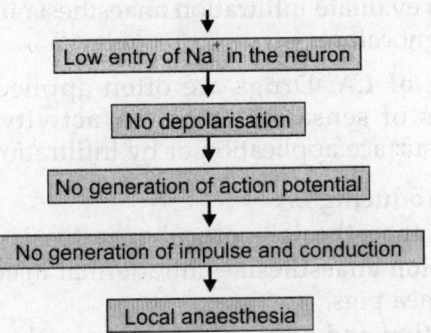

Combination of Vasoconstrictor with Local Anaesthetics

Advantages

1. Slow absorption from local site which results in prolonged duration of action of anaesthesia.
2. Less bleeding in surgical field.
3. Slow absorption of LA reduces systemic toxicity.

Disadvantages

1. Some parts of body like toes, ear lobule, tip of nose supplied by end arteries, adrenaline should not be used as vasoconstrictor, may lead to gangrene formation.
2. Absorption of adrenaline can cause systemic toxicity like tachycardia, palpitation and arrhythmia.
3. May delay wound healing by reducing blood supply to affected area.

Range

1:80,000–1:2,00,000—for dilution.

Side Effects

1. **CNS:** Initially CNS stimulation followed by depression that is restlessness, tremor, headache, drowsiness, confusion, convulsions followed by respiratory depression.
2. **CVS:** Bradycardia, hypotension, arrhythmia.
3. **Allergic reaction:** Skin rashes, itching, urticaria, sneezing, anaphylactic reaction.

Object: To evaluate infiltration anaesthesia in rabbit by 2% xylocaine (lignocaine).

Screening of LA: Drugs are often applied topically to produce loss of sensation, thus LA activity can be seen clinically by surface application or by infiltration.

Method of producing LA

1. **Surface anaesthesia**—corneal anaesthesia in rabbit.
2. **Infiltration anaesthesia**—intradermal injection in rabbit and guinea pigs.
3. **Conduction and nerve blocking anaesthesia in frog.**
4. **Spinal anaesthesia in dog.**

Infiltration anaesthesia: This experiment is carried out in guinea pig or rabbit. Clean the skin surface of the back side with 90% alcohol and allow to dry. Then 0.1 ml of lignocaine injected intradermally, raise a wheal around injected area. On another side give normal saline. After injection mark the margin of surrounding area with pen, pencil, and lightly prick the area with pin and repeat it at intervals.

S. No.	Time (min)	Response in TEST area	Response in CONTROL
1.	5	+	–
2.	10	+	–
3.	15	–	–
4.	20	–	–
5.	25	–	–
6.	30	–	–

Result

Absence of response in test area shows local anaesthetic property of lignocaine.

Experiment

To demonstrate analgesic activity of drugs by tail-flick method

Here the analgesic activity is estimated by an analgesiometer.

• Take two rats.
• Place one rat in rat holder, keeping the tail out.

- Now place tail tip in groove above the nichrome wire of analgesiometer.
- Switch on the analgesiometer, temperature in nichrome wire starts increasing. As the temperature increases, rat lifts the tail (tail flick) within 3–8 seconds. If tail takes more time, the animal is not suitable for experiment, and even skin can burn.
- Take two readings after 10 minutes gap and note the reaction time (control).
- Repeat the experiment after injecting morphine HCl 5 mg/kg intraperitoneal.
- Follow the same procedure in other in rat before and after injecting morphine HCl 10 mg/kg IP.
- Tabulate your finding.

Other Methods

1. Eddy's hot plate method
2. Writing test

Object: To study analgesic effect of morphine in rats by using tail-flick method.

Analgesia: It is defined as state of reduced awareness to pain.

Analgesics: Analgesics are substance which decreases pain sensation by increasing threshold to painful stimuli.

They can be divided into two groups:

I. Opioid/narcotic/morphine like analgesics.
II. Non-opioid/non-narcotic/aspirin like/antipyretic or anti-inflammatory analgesics.

Painful stimuli can be of three types:

Thermal: Radiant heat as a source of pain.

Chemical: Irritants like bradykinin and acetic acid.

Physical: Tail compression.

Commonly used method for evaluating analgesic activity of drug is:

1. Tail-flick method using analgesiometer (tail withdrawl from radiant heat).
2. Eddy's hot plate at 55°C (jumping from hot plate).

3. Hollander's method, pain by mechanical pressure.
4. Aconitin-induced writhing reflex to test NSAIDs activity.

Tail-flick method is based on the principle of thermal radiant heat and used for evaluation of centrally acting analgesics so this method can be used to differentiate between centrally acting opioids and non-opioids.

Procedure: Animal is placed in restrainer leaving the tail exposed outside the restrainer. Clean the tail with cotton with water or ethanol, leave the tail for drying, also give time for animal to settle down. Restrainer is now kept on analgesio-meter with proximal one-third of the tail is left because this portion is thick and keratinized. Keep the distal tail on the place made for tail above hot nichrome wire of analgesiometer, time of tail flick is noted. Screening is done before experiment. Rat showing reaction time more than 10 seconds and mice showing reaction time more than 6 seconds are excluded.

Analgesiometer: Here heated nichrome wire is used for producing pain in rat and mice tail. The temperature of wire is kept constant. Analgesic effect is measured by determining the reaction time of animal before and after administration of drugs.

Centrally acting analgesic increase reaction time: Drug used is morphine sulphate at dose of 5 mg/kg of body weight given intraperitoneally (IP). **Record your observation and make the observation table with results.**

QUESTIONS

Q 1. **What do you understand by local anaesthesia? Enumerate some methods of producing local anaesthesia.**

Q 2. **What are the advantages and disadvantages of combining adrenaline with local anaesthetic?**

Q 3. **What is the mechanism of local anaesthetic action?**

Q 4. **What are the methods for screening of local anaesthetics in experimental animals?**

Q 5. **What are the methods for screening of analgesics in experimental animals?**

13

Graph and Charts for Revision

Chart 13.1: Rabbit eye

Parameter	0 min		5 min		10 min	
	C	T	C	T	C	T
Pupil size (mm)	6	6	6	5	6	4
Light reflex	+	+	+	+	+	+
Corneal reflex	+	+	+	+	+	+
State of conjunctiva	P	P	P	C	P	C
(P = pale/c =congested)			(C= control eye, T = test eye)			

Q 1. Identify test drug (T).
Q 2. What precautions are necessary for this experiment?
Q 3. What are the ophthalmic uses of this drug?

Chart 13.2: Rabbit eye

Parameter	0 min		5 min		10 min	
	C	T	C	T	C	T
Light reflex	+	+	+	+	+	+
Corneal reflex	+	+	+	−	+	−
Pupil size (mm)	6	6	6	7	6	8
State of conjunctiva	P	P	P	P	P	P

Q 1. Identify drug (T).
Q 2. What is the mechanism of action of this drug?
Q 3. Describe the afferent and efferent pathway of corneal reflex.

Chart 13.3: Rabbit eye

Parameter	0 min		5 min		10 min	
	C	T	C	T	C	T
Pupil size (mm)	6	6	6	8	6	8
Light reflex	+	+	+	−	+	−
Corneal reflex	+	+	+	+	+	+
Conjunctival vessels	P	P	P	P	P	P
(P = pale)						

Q 1. Identify test drug (T).
Q 2. What are the ocular (ophthalmic) uses of this drug?
Q 3. What is active and passive mydriasis?

Chart 13.4: Rabbit eye

Parameter	0 min		5 min		10 min	
	C	T	C	T	C	T
Pupil size (mm)	6	6	6	7	6	7
Light reflex	+	+	+	+	+	+
Corneal reflex	+	+	+	+	+	+
Conjunctival vessels	P	P	P	P	P	P

Q 1. Identify the test drug (T).

Q 2. Name one mydriatic that does not cause cycloplegia.

Q 3. Name some drugs that decrease intraocular tension.

Graph 13.1: Blood pressure tracing of dog

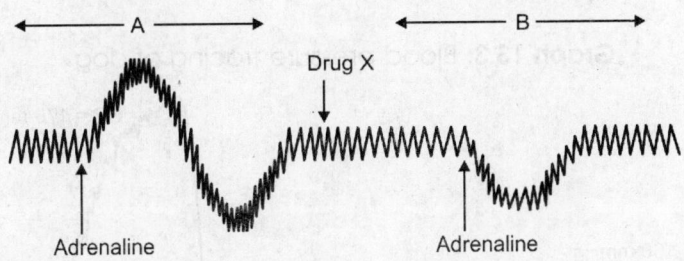

Q 1. Identify drug X.

Q 2. Effect of adrenaline on dog BP, i.e. segment A is also known as ———.

Q 3. Segment B is known as ——— and it is due to blockade of ———receptors.

Graph 13.2: Effect of drug on BP of dog

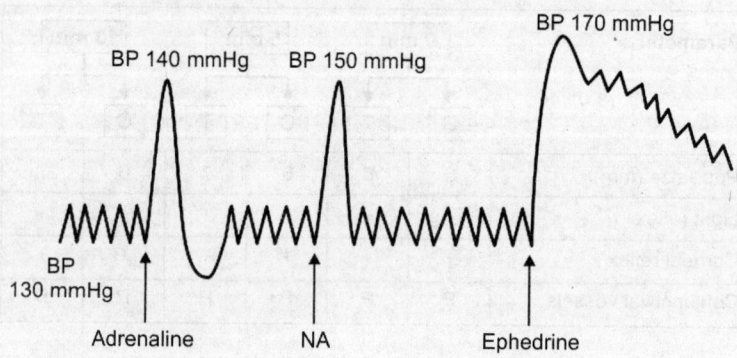

Q 1. Explain Graph 13.2.

Q 2. Explain the effect of drug—adrenaline, noradrenaline and ephedrine.

Q 3. Fall of BP after initial rise is seen in adrenaline but not with noradrenaline. Why?

Q 4. What is the difference between the effect of adrenaline and ephedrine?

Graph 13.3: Blood pressure tracing of dog

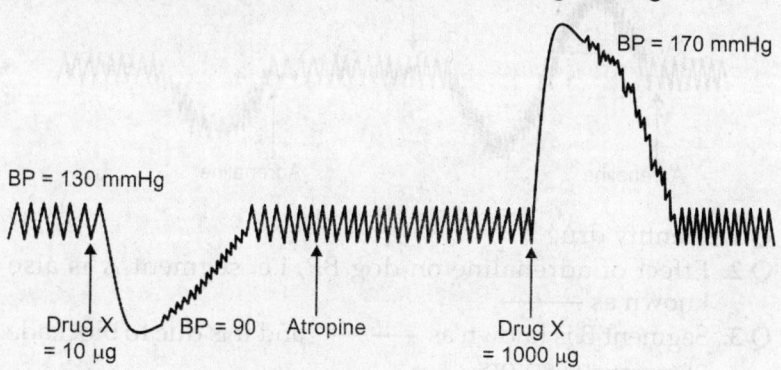

Q 1. Identify drug X.

Q 2. High dose (100 times) of drug (X) produced high BP and tachycardia. Explain it.

Q 3. What do you mean by ganglionic action of acetylcholine?

Graph 13.4: Blood pressure tracing of dog

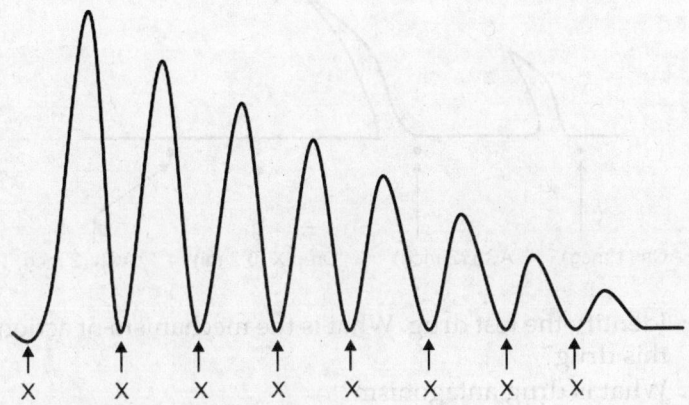

Q 1. This phenomenon is known as ——— .
Q 2. Drug X is ——— .
Q 3. What is the reason/mechanism behind this phenomenon?

Graph 13.5: Blood pressure tracing of dog

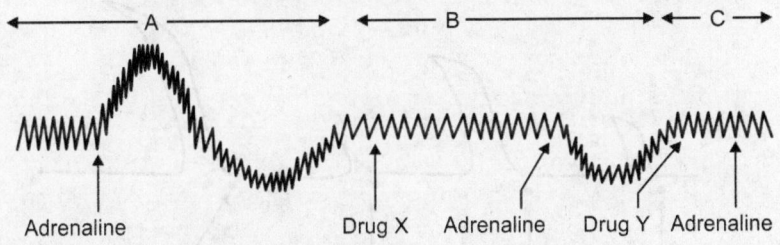

Q 1. Identify drug X and drug Y.
Q 2. Segments A, B and C are also known as ——— .
Q 3. Mention the receptors on which these drugs act:
    I. Adrenaline
    II. Noradrenaline
    III. Dopamine
    IV. Dobutamine
    V. Isoprenaline

Graph 13.6: Frog rectus

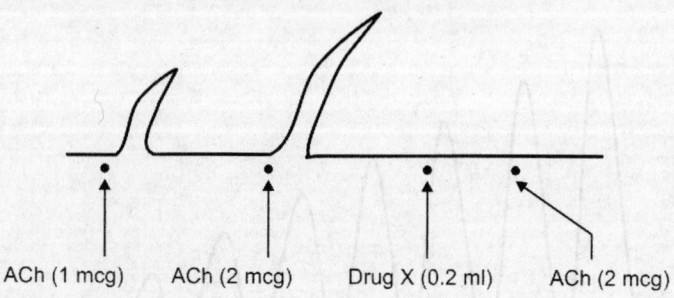

ACh (1 mcg)   ACh (2 mcg)   Drug X (0.2 ml)   ACh (2 mcg)

Q 1. Identify the test drug. What is the mechanism of action of this drug?

Q 2. What is drug antagonism?

Graph 13.7: Frog rectus

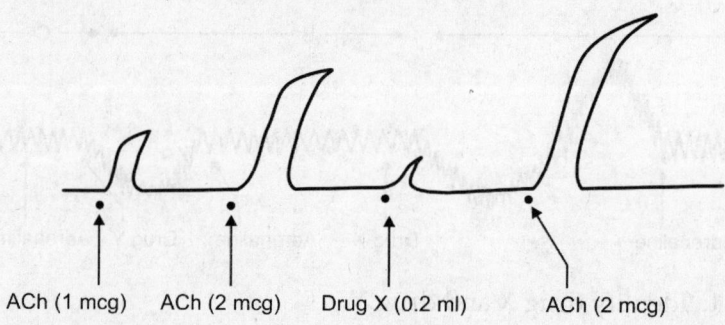

ACh (1 mcg)   ACh (2 mcg)   Drug X (0.2 ml)   ACh (2 mcg)

Q 1. Identify the test drug (X). What is the mechanism of action of this drug?

Q 2. What is potentiation?

Graph 13.8: Rabbit ileum experiment

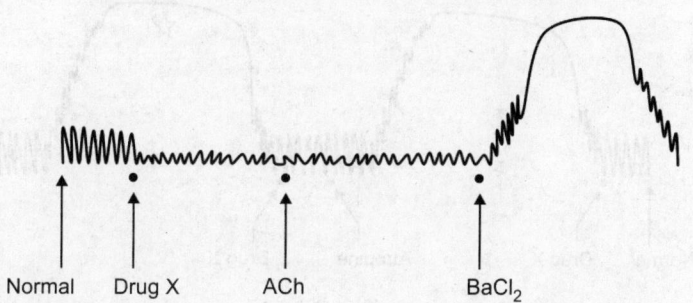

Normal   Drug X   ACh $BaCl_2$

Q 1. Identify the drug X.

Q 2. What is the mechanism of action of X?

Q 3. Acetylcholine is unable to show its effect but $BaCl_2$ can. Explain it.

Graph 13.9: Rabbit ileum

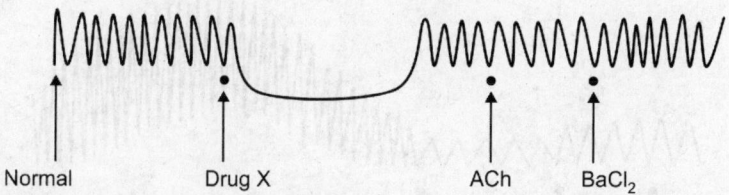

Normal   Drug X   ACh $BaCl_2$

Q 1. Identify the drug X.

Q 2. Comment on the mechanism and site of action of drug X.

Q 3. Name the PSS used in this experiment.

Graph 13.10: Rabbit ileum

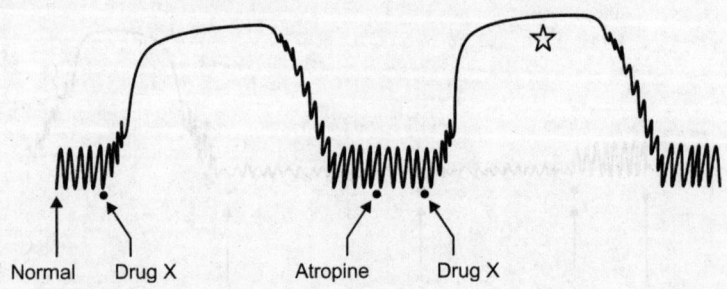

Q 1. Identify the drug X.
Q 2. Comment on the mechanism of action of drug X.
Q 3. Which type of contraction is produced by drug X?

Graph 13.11: Rabbit gut

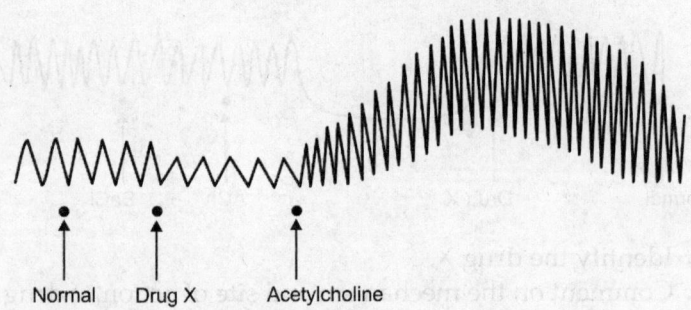

Q 1. Name the PSS and lever used in this experiment.
Q 2. Identify the drug X.
Q 3. Comment on the nature and site of action of drug X.

Graph 13.12: Rabbit gut

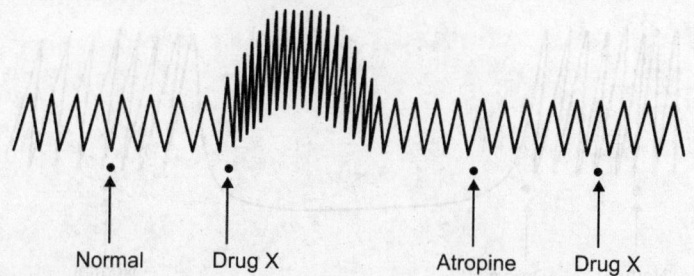

Normal   Drug X   Atropine   Drug X

Q 1. Name the PSS and lever used in this experiment.

Q 2. What is magnification in lever?

Q 3. Identify the drug X. What is the mechanism of action of drug X?

Graph 13.13: Frog heart

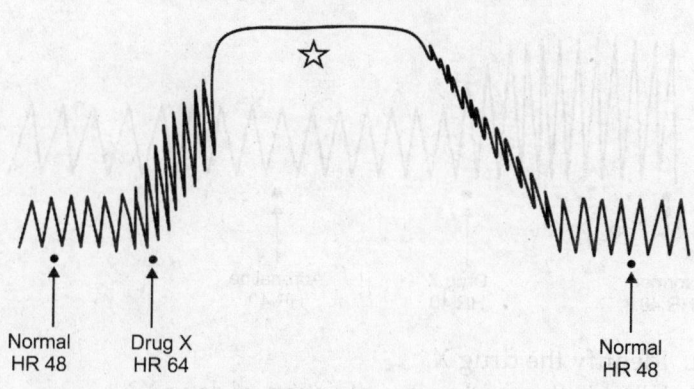

Normal   Drug X   Normal
HR 48   HR 64   HR 48

Q 1. Identify the drug X.

Q 2. What is the mechanism of action of drug X?

Q 3. Which type of arrest is produced by this drug?

Graph 13.14: Frog heart

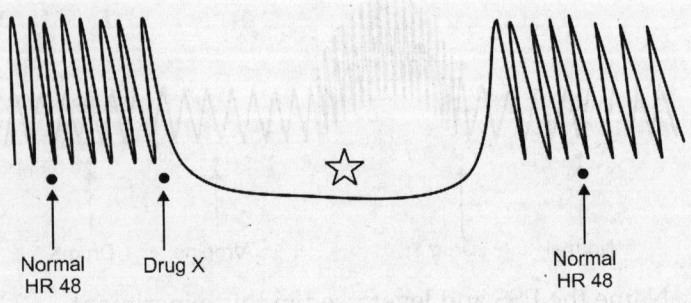

Normal
HR 48

Drug X

Normal
HR 48

Q 1. Identify the drug X.
Q 2. What is the mechanism of action of drug X?
Q 3. Which type of arrest is produced by this drug?

Graph 13.15: Cardiac stimulants and depressants

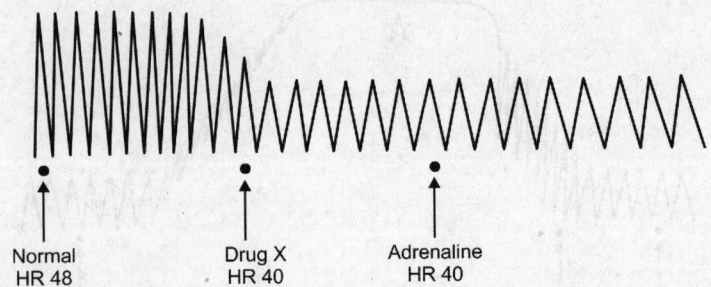

Normal
HR 48

Drug X
HR 40

Adrenaline
HR 40

Q 1. Identify the drug X.
Q 2. What is the mechanism of action of drug X?
Q 3. What is drug antagonism?

Graph 13.16: Cardiac stimulants and depressants

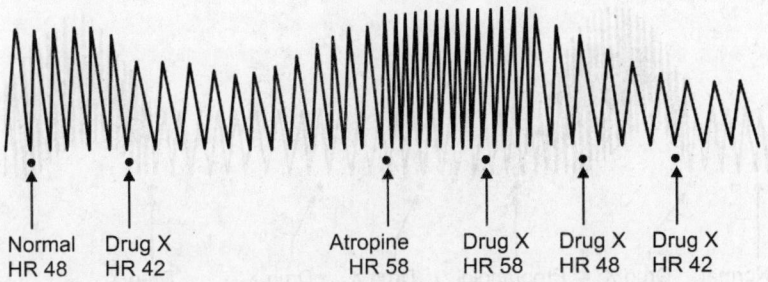

Normal HR 48 Drug X HR 42 Atropine HR 58 Drug X HR 58 Drug X HR 48 Drug X HR 42

Q 1. Name the PSS and lever used in this experiment.

Q 2. Identify the drug X.

Q 3. Comment on the type of antagonism shown in this graph.

Graph 13.17: Cardiac stimulants and depressants

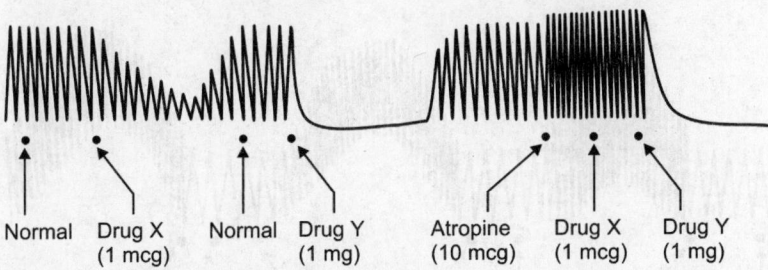

Normal Drug X (1 mcg) Normal Drug Y (1 mg) Atropine (10 mcg) Drug X (1 mcg) Drug Y (1 mg)

Q 1. Identify the drugs X and Y.

Q 2. Comment on the nature and site of action of drugs X and Y.

Q 3. What is magnification in lever?

Graph 13.18: Cardiac stimulants and depressants

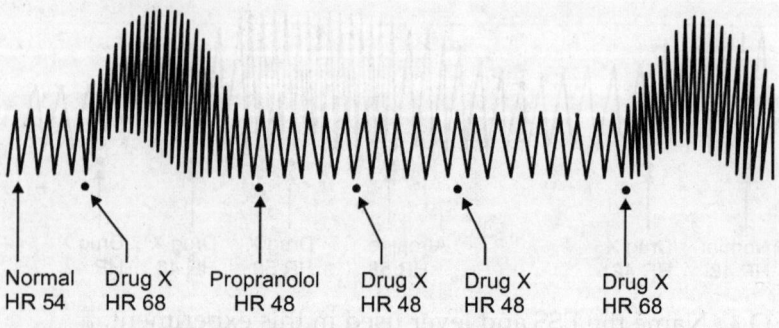

Normal   Drug X   Propranolol   Drug X   Drug X   Drug X
HR 54   HR 68   HR 48   HR 48   HR 48   HR 68

Q 1. Identify the drug X.

Q 2. What is the mechanism of drug X?

Q 3. Which type of antagonism is shown by drug X in this graph?

Graph 13.19: Frog heart

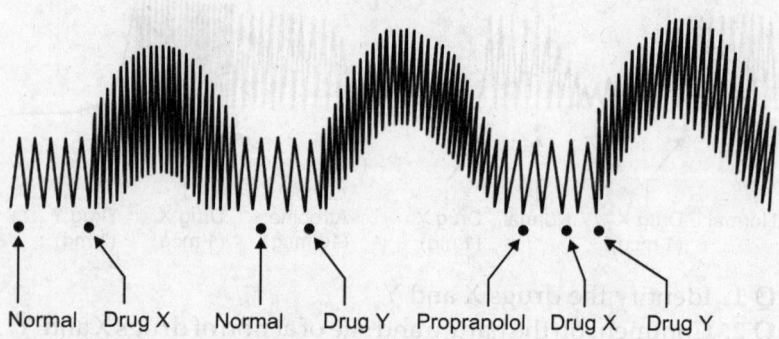

Normal   Drug X   Normal   Drug Y   Propranolol   Drug X   Drug Y

Q 1. Identify the drugs X and Y.

Q 2. The drug X is unable to produce its response but drug Y can, after giving the blocker. Explain it.

Q 3. Name cardiac stimulants and depressants.

Graph 13.20: Dose response curve

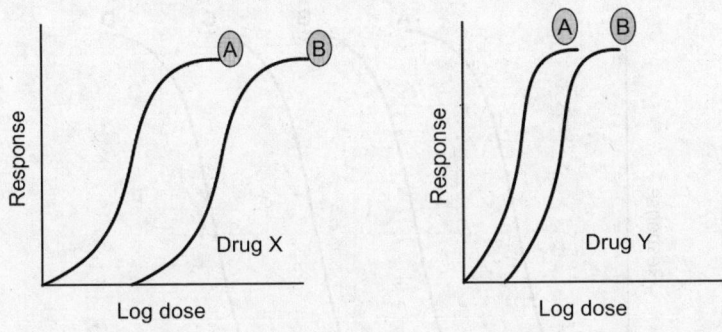

The therapeutic and adverse effect of two drugs "X" and "Y" is shown in curves in "A" and "B" respectively.

Q. Comment on therapeutic index safety and toxicity profile.

Graph 13.21: Dose response curve

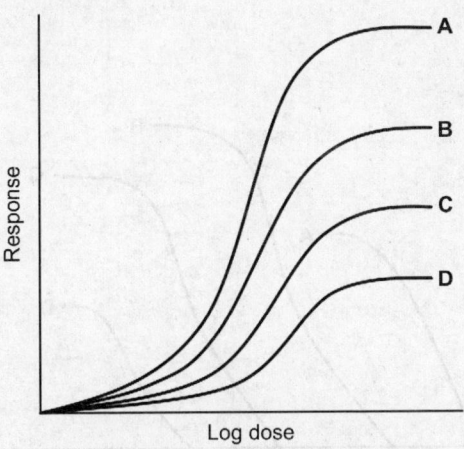

Q. Comment on type of drug antagonism in dose response curve.

Graph 13.22: Dose response curve

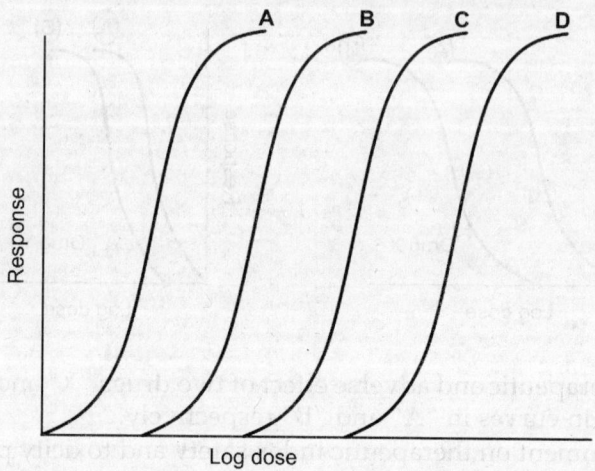

Q. Comment on type of drug antagonism in dose response curve.

Graph 13.23: Dose response curve

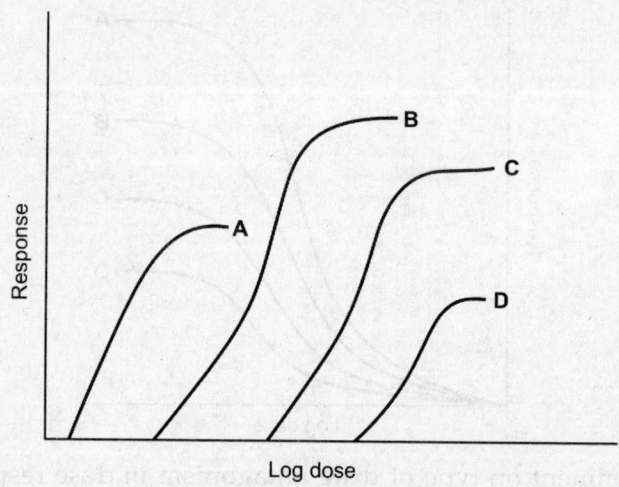

Q 1. Comment on efficacy and potency.
Q 2. Which drug is most potent in this DRC?

14

Viva Voce Questions in Experimental Pharmacology

1. What do you understand by experimental pharmacology?
2. What are the aims of experimental pharmacology?
3. What do you understand by pharmacokinetics?
4. What do you understand by pharmacodynamics?
5. What do you understand by *in vivo, in vitro* and *in silico* study?
6. Name some common laboratory animals used in experiments.
7. What do you understand by nude mice?
8. What do you understand by knockout mice?
9. Name two strains of albino rats used in experiments.
10. Tail-flick method is used for screening of which type of activity?
11. To study the effect of histamine on ileum, which experimental animal should be preferred?
12. For demonstration of Dale's vasomotor reversal, which animal is used?
13. Comment on rat as experimental animal.
14. Comment on rabbit as experimental animal.
15. What are the physical and chemical methods of euthanasia?
16. What do you understand by CPCSEA?
17. Name some commonly used instruments in experimental pharmacology.

18. Who first designed commonly used organ bath?
19. What precautions should be kept in mind while mounting the isolated tissue such as rectus abdominis or ileum?
20. When the maintenance of temperature of organ bath is required?
21. Define PSS.
22. Name some common PSS and their uses.
23. Give the composition of frog Ringer solution.
24. Give the composition of Tyrode solution.
25. In which experiments, frog Ringer solution is used as PSS?
26. In which experiments, Tyrode solution is used as PSS?
27. What do you understand by tone, amplitude and rate?
28. Give one example of type 1 and type 2 lever used in experiments.
29. Give one example of isometric and isotonic lever.
30. What do you understand by magnification in mechanical levers?
31. In which type of experiments frontal writing lever is used?
32. In which type of experiments Starling's lever is used?
33. What do you understand by receptor?
34. What are the differences between agonist, antagonist, inverse agonist and partial agonist?
35. Give two examples of GPCRs.
36. Give two examples of ligand gated ion channels.
37. Comment about cholinoceptors.
38. Comment about adrenergic receptors.
39. What do you understand by presynaptic and postsynaptic receptors?
40. What do you understand by autoreceptors and hetero-receptors?
41. What do you understand by downregulation and upregulation of receptors.
42. What is the difference between dose response curve and log dose response curve?
43. What are the advantages of log dose response curve?
44. What information can be derived from a log dose response curve?
45. Define potency and efficacy.

46. How can we compare the potency and efficacy of two drugs from their log dose response curves?
47. In graded DRC, what do you understand by ceiling response?
48. Define tolerance. What change will occur in DRC?
49. What do you understand by potentiation and antagonism?
50. What are the different types of receptor antagonism? Give one example of each.
51. What do you understand by therapeutic index?
52. Among benzodiazepines and barbiturates, which one have a high therapeutic index?
53. What do you understand by bioassay?
54. What are the indications of bioassay?
55. What are the types of bioassay?
56. What do you understand by quantal bioassay?
57. What do you understand by graded response bioassay?
58. What do you understand by matching assay?
59. What do you understand by three-point assay?
60. What do you understand by bracketing assay?
61. What are the advantages and disadvantages of three-point assay?
62. What is the preferred tissue for bioassay of histamine?
63. What do you understand by ceiling response in a log dose response curve?
64. What information can be derived from a log dose response curve?
65. What are the advantages of sigmoid log dose response curve?
66. Name some spasmogenic and spasmolytics used in rabbit ileum experiment.
67. What is the action of acetylcholine, atropine and adrenaline on GIT?
68. What is the action of Barium chloride and papaverine on GIT?
69. Name the parameters that we study in the graph of rabbit gut experiment.

70. In rabbit ileum experiment, what should be the ideal temperature of organ bath and why?
71. Name the PSS, its composition and lever used in rabbit ileum experiment.
72. Which part of gut is selected in rabbit gut experiment and why?
73. What is the effect of adrenaline and atropine on tone and amplitude of in rabbit ileum experiment?
74. What is the effect of barium chloride and papaverine on tone and amplitude in rabbit ileum experiment?
75. Name two spasmolytic drugs and their indications.
76. Why movements of ileum are recorded even when the nerve supply is cut?
77. How will you establish the site of action of spasmogenic drug in rabbit ileum experiment?
78. How will you establish the site of action of spasmolytic drug in rabbit ileum experiment?
79. Name the receptors involved in action of acetylcholine, atropine and adrenaline in GIT.
80. How much magnification is needed in rabbit ileum experiment?
81. Name two miotics and two mydriatics used in rabbit eye experiment.
82. What is the mechanism behind miosis and mydriasis?
83. What do you understand by active and passive mydriasis? Name one drug that produces it.
84. What do you understand by active and passive miosis? Name one drug that produces it.
85. Which receptors are involved in sphincter pupillae and dilator pupillae action in eye?
86. What are the ocular effects of cholinomimetics?
87. What are the ocular effects of antimuscarinic drug atropine?
88. What are the ocular effects of sympathomimetics?
89. What are the ocular effects of local anaesthetics?
90. What parameters we study in rabbit eye experiment?
91. Differentiate active and passive miosis.
92. Differentiate active and passive mydriasis.

93. What is the afferent and efferent pathway in light reflex?
94. Name one drug that causes abolition of light reflex.
95. Name one drug that causes abolition of corneal reflex.
96. Name one drug that causes increased vascularity of conjunctival blood vessels.
97. Name one drug that causes increased intraocular tension.
98. Name some drugs that cause decreased intraocular tension.
99. What precautions are necessary in rabbit eye experiment?
100. What do you understand by cycloplegia? Name a drug that produces cycloplegia.
101. Name a mydriatic that is not a cycloplegic.
102. What are the ocular uses of miotics?
103. What are the ocular uses of mydriatics?
104. What are the important anatomical and physiological features of frog heart?
105. Name some cardiac stimulants and cardiac depressants used in isolated and perfused frog heart experiment.
106. Name the adrenergic and cholinergic receptors of heart.
107. What are the cardiac effects of cholinomimetics?
108. What are the cardiac effects of atropine?
109. What are the cardiac effects of adrenaline?
110. What are the cardiac effects of potassium chloride and calcium chloride?
111. What are the cardiac effects of low dose and high dose calcium chloride?
112. What do you understand by systolic arrest? Name a drug producing it.
113. What do you understand by diastolic arrest? Name a drug producing it.
114. Name the PSS used in isolated and perfused frog heart experiment and its composition.
115. How will you establish the site of action of cardiac stimulants in isolated and perfused frog heart experiment?
116. How will you establish the site of action of cardiac depressants in isolated and perfused frog heart experiment?

117. What do you understand by reversible competitive antagonism? Explain it by one example in frog heart experiment.
118. Name the anaesthetic used in dog BP experiment.
119. Which artery and vein is utilized for measuring BP and injecting drugs in dog BP experiment?
120. What do you understand by biphasic response of adrenaline on BP?
121. Explain the Dale's vasomotor reversal phenomenon.
122. Mention the receptors on which adrenaline acts.
123. Mention the receptors on which noradrenaline acts.
124. Mention the receptors on which isoprenaline acts.
125. What are the differences in the cardiovascular actions of adrenaline and noradrenaline?
126. What are the differences in the cardiovascular actions of acetylcholine and isoprenaline?
127. What are the differences in the cardiovascular actions of adrenaline and ephedrine?
128. Biphasic response and Dale's reversal is not seen in case of noradrenaline. Why?
129. What are the cardiovascular actions of atropine?
130. What are the cardiovascular actions of propranolol?
131. What are the cardiovascular actions of phentolamine?
132. What do you understand by ganglionic action of acetylcholine, how will you elicit it?
133. What do you understand by tachyphylaxis?
134. What is the difference between tolerance and tachyphylaxis?
135. What is the mechanism of tachyphylaxis?

15

Effect of Drugs on Rabbit's Eye

Objective: To demonstrate the effect of miotic, mydriatic and local anaesthetic on various parameters in rabbit eye. Write down the objective, required materials, procedures and precautions of this experiment. Tabulate your observations and write down your inference.

Materials Required
- Rabbit, rabbit holder, dropper, torch, cotton wisp, measuring scale, Tonopen.
- Drugs and solutions.
- Normal saline (0.9%), physostigmine (0.5%), pilocarpine (1%), atropine (1%), phenylephrine (5%), lignocaine (1%).

Procedure
1. Hold the rabbit by its ears with one hand while supporting its bottom with the other hand.
2. Fix the rabbit in rabbit holder.
3. Clip the eyelashes using the curved scissors since the eyelashes may interfere while administering drugs and eliciting the corneal reflex.
4. Take care not to injure the eyes or eyelids of rabbit.
5. Keep one eye (either left or right eye) as control and other as test.
6. Use normal saline as control.

7. Wash thoroughly to remove the residual drugs, if any instilled before.
8. Use pouch technique to instill the drugs in the eye.
9. Press the medial canthus for a minute, after instilling the drug so that the drug does not escape through nasolacrimal duct.
10. Measure/elicit the following parameters in both control and drug treated eyes and tabulate the readings
    - Light reflex = present (+) or absent (−)
    - Corneal reflex = present (+) or absent (−)
    - Diameter of pupils (in mm) = (horizontal diameter + vertical diameter)/2
    - Intraocular tension (mmHg)

Precautions

- Keep the rabbit in dimly-lit room.
- Discard the animal if it has conjunctivitis, uveitis, etc.
- Discard drugs if discolored or expired.
- Follow aseptic precautions while instilling the drug. The tip of the dropper should not touch the eye.
- Do not instill more than 2–3 drops of a drug.
- Use fresh rabbit to test each drug.
- Both the eyes must be thoroughly washed with normal saline to remove the residual drugs.
- Use scale provided to measure the pupil size. Each division is 1 mm.
- Reassure the animal by gently patting/stroking its back, if it is agitated or aggressive.

Experiment on computer

1. Click on the cage for a fresh rabbit.
2. Drag it to rabbit holder.
3. Adjust the ambient light of room and click to have a closer view.
4. Select one eye (usually left eye) as control and the other eye as test eye.
5. Instill normal saline in control eye and drug in test eye.
6. Zoom in for a closer view.

7. Observe:
   - Light reflex = present (+) or absent (–)
   - Corneal reflex = present (+) or absent (–)
   - Pupil size = (horizontal diameter + vertical diameter)/2
   - IOP = measured with tonopen (mmHg)
8. Wash both the eyes with normal saline.
9. Take a fresh rabbit for each drug
   - Diameter of the pupil is measured with a scale measure: Horizontal and vertical diameter, add them and divide it by two.
   - The light reflex is elicited by focusing light from a torch into the eye from one side. It leads to pupillary constriction in both eyes. The eye in which light was shown is direct and the other one is indirect (consensual).

Observations: Rabbit eye experiment on CAL

Rabbit	Eye	Drug (mm)	Pupil size			LR (+/−)		CR (+/−)		IOP (mm Hg)		
			B	A	D	B	A	B	A	B	A	D
1.	Test control	Pilocarpine NS/DW										
2.	Test control	Physostigmine NS/DW										
3.	Test control	Phenylephrine NS/DW										
4.	Test control	Atropine NS/DW										
5.	Test control	Lignocaine NS/DW										

LR = light reflex
CR = corneal reflex
B = before
A = after
D = difference
NS/DW = normal saline/distilled water
(+) = present
(–) = abolished

- The corneal reflex is tested by touching the corneo-scleral junction with a piece of cotton each time from side leads to blink response.
- Intraocular pressure is measured with a tonometer adapted for rabbit eyes.

Discussion

Ocular effects and clinical importance of miotics, mydriatics and local anaesthetics

1. **Miotics:** Pilocarpine (0.5–4%) eye drops, also available as ocusert and physostigmine (0.1–1.0%). Pilocarpine is directly acting cholinomimetic (M3 muscarinic action) while physostigmine is indirectly acting cholinomimetic (reversible anticholinesterase). They act on muscarinic receptors of sphincter pupillae (= circular) muscles of iris producing pupillary constriction (= active miosis). Contraction of ciliary body by miotics leads to better aqueous outflow because of opening of trabecular meshwork, and spasm of accommodation because of more spherical shape of lens produced by relaxation of suspensory ligaments (=zonules) and eye is accommodated for near vision. They also produce lacrimation due to stimulation of M3 receptors at lacrimal glands. IOP (intraocular pressure) falls (especially in glaucomatous patients with iridocorneal angle closure) because of better drainage of aqueous humour through the removal of pupillary block. They are not preferred in open angle glaucoma because of several drawbacks (decreased pupil size, diminution of vision, headache, brow pain). Alpha adrenergic receptor antagonists (alpha blockers) produce passive miosis (because of blockade of action of radial = dilator pupillae muscle of iris having α_1 receptors, and subsequent unopposed action of circular = sphincter pupillae muscle of iris). But alpha blockers are not classified or used as ocular miotics.

2. **Mydriatics:** These drugs produce pupillary dilatation. Two groups of drugs are classified as mydriatics:
   a. Atropine (muscarinic receptor antagonist) and atropine substitutes (homatropine, cyclopentolate, tropicamide)

b. Alpha-adrenergic receptor agonist (= sympatho-mimetic), e.g. phenylephrine.

Ocular effects of antimuscarinic drugs include passive mydriasis (because of blockade of action of sphincter pupillae and subsequent unopposed action of dilator pupillae), abolished light reflex, photophobia and cycloplegia (paralysis of accommodation) due to blockade of muscarinic receptors at ciliary body (suspensory ligaments become tightened and lens become less spherical and eye is fixed at distant vision). The eyes become dry due to decreased lacrimation (blockade of M3 receptor at lacrimal glands). The chief disadvantage of atropine is longer duration of action, so cycloplegia lasts for a week. Mydriasis can precipitate the rise of IOP (mydriasis result in reduced drainage of aqueous humour due to blockade of canal of Schlemm by falling of iris over the canal) especially in elderly individuals or in persons with shallow anterior chamber or narrow iridocorneal angle, so atropinic drugs are contraindicated in patients of glaucoma. For mydriatic effect atropine substitutes with shorter duration of action and lesser cycloplegia, e.g. tropicamide is preferred in adults.

Another group of mydriatics include sympathomi-metics, e.g. phenylephrine, which produce active mydriasis (due to contraction of dilator pupillae muscles of iris having α_1 receptors). They neither affect light reflex nor they produce cycloplegia. They tend to reduce IOP due to decreased aqueous secretion.

Ocular indications for mydriatics
   i. Determination of refractive error (both mydriasis and cycloplegia is needed)
  ii. Fundus examination
 iii. Breaking the adhesions formed between lens and cornea or iris, in iridocyclitis (mydriatics are alter-nated with the miotics).
  iv. Treatment of iritis, iridocyclitis, keratitis, choroiditis (atropine is preferred due to long-lasting action and anodyne = pain relieving effect).

3. Local anaesthetics: Lignocaine and cocaine produce corneal anaesthesia so loss of corneal reflex. Lignocaine produces no change on pupil size or IOP, while cocaine produces mydriasis and sympathomimetic effects (due to inhibition of reuptake of catecholamines) along with rise of IOP. Light reflex remains unaffected.

Local anaesthetics, e.g. tetracaine (1–2%), proparacaine (0.5–1%), lignocaine (2–5%) are used topically for surface anaesthesia in eye for:

  i. Removal of ocular foreign body
 ii. Infiltration and retrobulbar anaesthesia
iii. Preoperative preparation
 iv. Prior to tonometry.

16

DRC of Acetylcholine on Frog's Rectus Abdominis Muscle

Objective: To record the dose response curve of acetylcholine on isolated frog rectus abdominis muscle. Write down the materials required and procedure of the experiment. Draw a schematic graph of DRC of acetylcholine based on your observation and write the inference.

- Materials required: Animal: Frog; PSS: Frog Ringer solution; Drug: Acetylcholine in different concentrations (10–400 microgram/ml). Instruments: Kymograph, student organ bath, aerator, insulin syringe, dissecting board and various dissecting instruments, sideway lever, plasticine, stopwatch, curved needle, thread, graph paper.
- Procedure

Dissection and Separation of Tissue (Fig.16.1)

1. Stunning of frog
2. Double pithing of frog
3. Pin four limbs on dissecting board, ventral part facing above
4. Remove abdominal skin and expose the rectus abdominis muscle
5. Take out muscle on dish with frog Ringer solution, spread gently

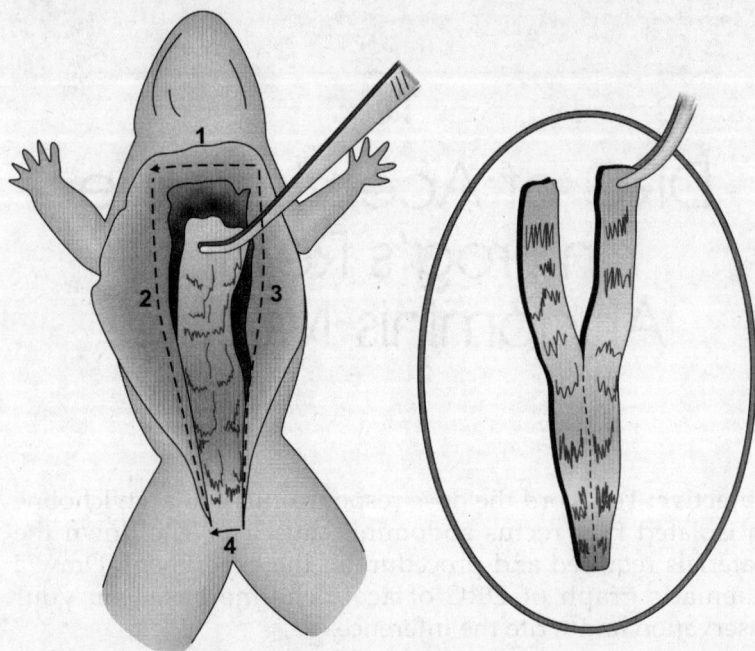

Fig. 16.1: Dissection and separation of rectus abdominis muscle in frog

Mounting of Tissue and Graph

- Cut into two longitudinal pieces and transfer one piece to **frog Ringer solution.**
- Thread is attached at each end of preparation.
- Preparation is mounted in organ bath of capacity **10–20 ml at room temperature.**
- **Contractions are recorded with a simple sideways-writing lever or frontal writing lever.**
- **The muscle should be kept for relaxation for 30–45 min by applying load of one gram using plasticine on the long side arm of the lever that must be equidistant from the fulcrum.**
- **Contractions are obtained by administrating drugs to the organ bath.**

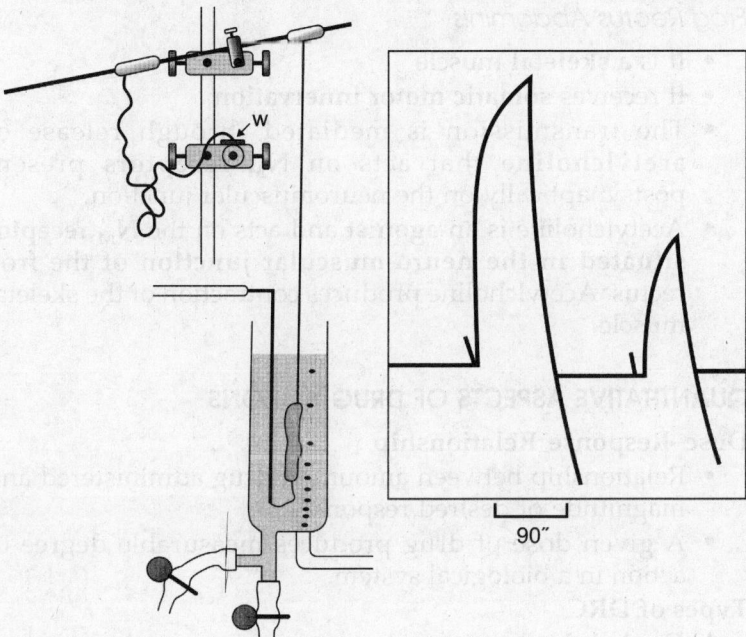

Fig. 16.2: Mounted rectus muscle in the organ bath and the response produced by it

Precautions

1. The level of PSS (Frog Ringer) in the inner organ bath should remain constant throughout the experiment, by marking the level with a marker.
2. The thread of the rectus muscle should not come in contact with the wall of organ bath.
3. A steady and constant stream of air should be passed in the organ bath to avoid tissue destruction.
4. There is no need to maintain the temperature of organ bath, since frog is cold-blooded animal, its temperature varies according to environmental temperature.
5. Drum speed is kept slow and the lever should be placed tangential to the drum.
6. Dose cycle is followed strictly (contact time = 90 seconds, rest for 3 wash and baseline of 45 seconds) (Fig.16.2)
7. Follow the sequence (baseline—inject the drug—wash).

Frog Rectus Abdominis
- It is a **skeletal** muscle
- It receives **somatic motor innervation**
- The transmission is mediated through release of **acetylcholine** that acts on N_M **receptors** present postsynaptically on the neuromuscular junction.
- Acetylcholine is an **agonist** and acts on the N_M **receptor situated in the neuro-muscular junction** of the frog rectus. Acetylcholine produces contraction of the skeletal muscle.

QUANTITATIVE ASPECTS OF DRUG ACTIONS

Dose–Response Relationship
- Relationship between amount of drug administered and magnitude of desired response.
- A given dose of drug produces measurable degree of action in a biological system.

Types of DRC
1. **Graded dose–response**
2. **Quantal dose–response**

Graded Dose–Response
- When dose of drug is increased, the response also increases till the maximum (= ceiling) response is achieved.
- Relationship between the dose and response can be plotted (x-axis = dose/concentration; y-axis = response)
- Concentration versus response on arithmetic scale, curve is *hyperbolic*.
- Concentration versus response on log scale, curve is *sigmoid-shaped.*

Advantages of Log DRC
1. The linear section of the sigmoid curve becomes straight.
2. Comparison of two DRCs is much simpler on log DRC.
3. Large dose ranges can be plotted.
- **Threshold dose:** The minimum dose of a drug which elicits biological response by the tissue.

- **Ceiling dose:** The minimum dose which elicits the maximum biological effect by the isolated tissue. The increment in the doses beyond the ceiling dose do not induce further increase in biological activity.
- **Experiment on CAL**
  1. Doses of acetylcholine are increased in a geometric progression (i.e. doubled), such as 0.05 ml, 0.1 ml, 0.2 ml, 0.4 ml, 0.8 ml, 1.6 ml, 3.2 ml, etc. [Fig. 16.3(a)]
  2. Record the responses till the maximum (= ceiling) response is achieved.

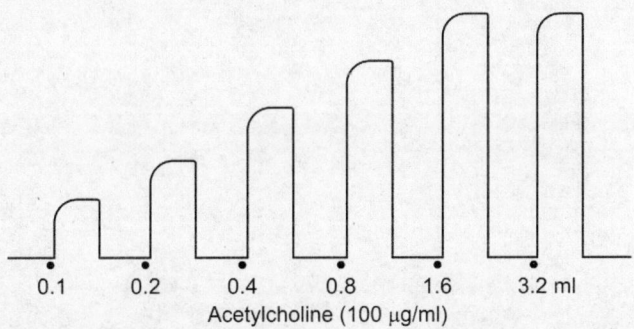

Fig. 16.3a: Graded responses to increase concentrations of acetylcholine

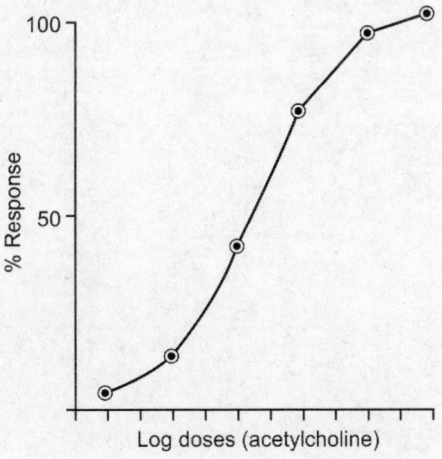

Fig. 16.3b: Log DRC of acetylcholine

3. Do not repeatedly expose the tissue to higher doses, once ceiling response is achieved (because the tissue become unresponsive).

4. Measure the height of responses in centimeter and the corresponding doses.

5. Plot the log DRC by plotting log doses on x-axis and percent of response on y-axis.

6. Explain the characteristics of the curve obtained [Fig. 16.3(b)].

17

Potentiation and Antagonism Effect on DRC of Acetylcholine

Objective: To record the dose response curve of acetylcholine in presence of (i) physostigmine and (ii) d-tubocurarine on isolated frog rectus abdominis muscle. Write down the materials required and procedure of the experiment. Draw a schematic graph of DRC of acetylcholine based on your observation and write the inference.

- Materials required: Animal: Frog; PSS: Frog Ringer solution; Drug: Acetylcholine in different concentrations (10–400 microgram/ml), Physostigmine (2 mg/ml), d-tubocurarine (2 mg/ml). Instruments: Kymograph, student organ bath, aerator, insulin syringe, dissecting board and various dissecting instruments, sideway lever, plasticine, stopwatch, curved needle, thread, graph paper.
- Procedure

Dissection and Separation of Tissue

1. Stunning of frog
2. Double pithing of frog
3. Pin four limbs on dissecting board, ventral part facing above
4. Remove abdominal skin and expose the rectus abdominis muscle
5. Take out muscle on dish with frog Ringer solution, spread gently

125

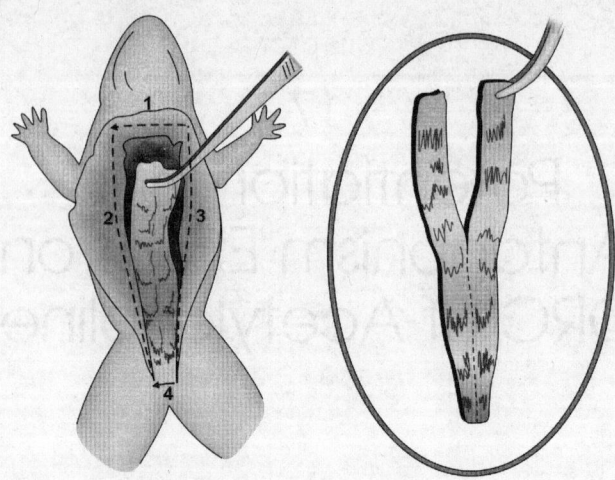

Fig. 17.1: Dissection and separation of rectus abdominis muscle in frog

Mounting of Tissue and Graph

- Cut into two longitudinal pieces and transfer one piece to **frog Ringer solution**.
- Thread is attached at each end of preparation.
- Preparation is mounted in organ-bath of capacity **10–20 ml at room temperature**.
- **Contractions are recorded with a simple sideways— writing lever or frontal writing lever.**
- **The muscle should be kept for relaxation for 30–45 min by applying load of one gram using plasticine on the long side arm of the lever that must be equidistant from the fulcrum.**
- **Contractions are obtained by administrating drugs to the organ bath**
  - i. Records the concentration–response curve of acetylcholine (10–400 µg/ml), starting from the minimum concentration till the ceiling response is achieved. Plot the log DRC of acetylcholine.
  - ii. Record the concentration-response curve of acetylcholine in the presence of physostigmine (2 mg/ml),

by adding physostigmine into the reservoir containing frog Ringer solution and irrigate the tissue with this mixed PSS for 30 min. **Plot the log DRC of acetylcholine in the presence of physostigmine.**

iii In another set-up or on different piece of rectus, add d-tubocurarine (2 mg/ml) to the reservoir containing frog Ringer solution (PSS) and irrigate the tissue for 30 min. **Plot the log DRC of acetylcholine in the presence of d-tubocurarine.**

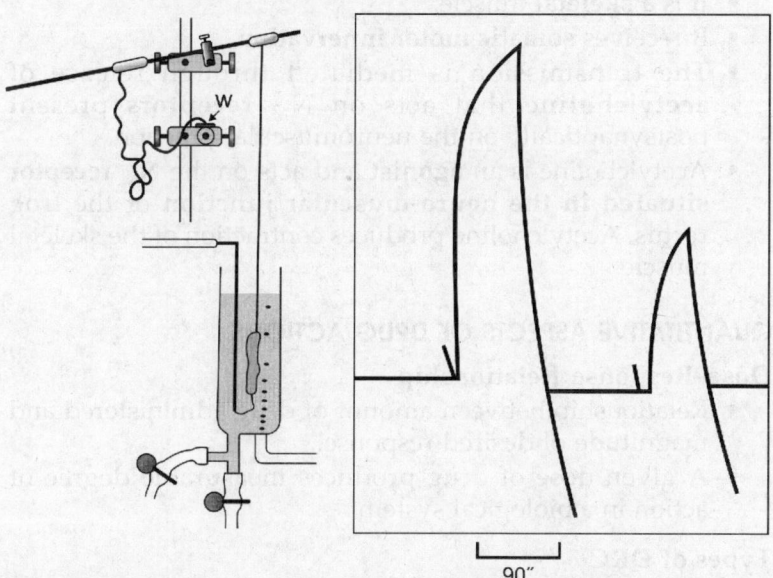

90″

Fig. 17.2: Mounted rectus muscle in the organ bath and the response produced by it

Precautions

1. The level of PSS (frog Ringer) in the inner organ bath should remain constant throughout the experiment, by marking the level with a marker.
2. The thread of the rectus muscle should not come in contact with the wall of organ bath.
3. A steady and constant stream of air should be passed in the organ bath to avoid tissue destruction.

4. There is no need to maintain the temperature of organ bath, since frog is cold-blooded animal, its temperature varies according to environmental temperature.
5. Drum speed is kept slow and the lever should be placed tangential to the drum.
6. Dose cycle is followed strictly (contact time= 90 seconds, rest for 3 wash and baseline of 45 seconds) (Fig. 17.2)
7. Follow the sequence (baseline—inject the drug—wash).

Frog Rectus Abdominis
- It is a **skeletal** muscle.
- It receives **somatic motor innervation**
- The transmission is mediated through release of **acetylcholine** that acts on N_M **receptors** present postsynaptically on the neuromuscular junction.
- Acetylcholine is an **agonist** and acts on the N_M **receptor situated in the neuro-muscular junction** of the frog rectus. Acetylcholine produces contraction of the skeletal muscle.

QUANTITATIVE ASPECTS OF DRUG ACTIONS
Dose–Response Relationship
- Relationship between amount of drug administered and magnitude of desired response.
- A given dose of drug produces measurable degree of action in a biological system.

Types of DRC
1. **Graded dose–response**
2. **Quantal dose–response**

Graded Dose–response
- When dose of drug is increased, the response also increases till the maximum (=ceiling) response is achieved.
- Relationship between the dose and response can be plotted (x-axis=dose/concentration; y-axis=response)
- Concentration versus response on arithmetic scale, curve is *hyperbolic*.

- Concentration versus response on log scale, curve is *sigmoid-shaped.*

Advantages of Log DRC

1. The linear section of the sigmoid curve becomes straight.
2. Comparison of two DRCs is much simpler on log DRC.
3. Large dose ranges can be plotted.

Threshold dose: The minimum dose of a drug which elicits biological response by the tissue.

Ceiling dose: The minimum dose which elicits the maximum biological effect by the isolated tissue. The increment in the doses beyond the ceiling dose does not induce further increase in biological activity.

- **Potentiating effect of Physostigmine:** After adding Physostigmine, the same dose of acetylcholine produces an increased response. The log DRC is shifted to left.
- Mechanism of action of physostigmine: It inhibits the cholinesterase enzyme, thereby *potentiates the effect of acetylcholine.* It is indirectly acting cholinergic drug.
- **Antagonism by d-tubocurarine:** d-TC is a neuro-muscular blocker that blocks the N_M receptors at NMJ of skeletal muscle (frog rectus abdominis). After adding d-TC, the same dose of acetylcholine produces a decreased response and log DRC is shifted to right. This is competitive antagonism, so the shift of the curve is parallel without the change of maximum response.
- **Experiment on CAL**
  1. Doses of acetylcholine is increased in a geometric progression (i.e. doubled), such as 0.05 ml, 0.1 ml, 0.2 ml, 0.4 ml, 0.8 ml, 1.6 ml, 3.2 ml, etc.
  2. Record the responses till the maximum (= ceiling) response is achieved.
  3. Do not repeatedly expose the tissue to higher doses, once ceiling response is achieved (because the tissue becomes unresponsive).
  4. Measure the height of responses in centimeter and the corresponding doses.

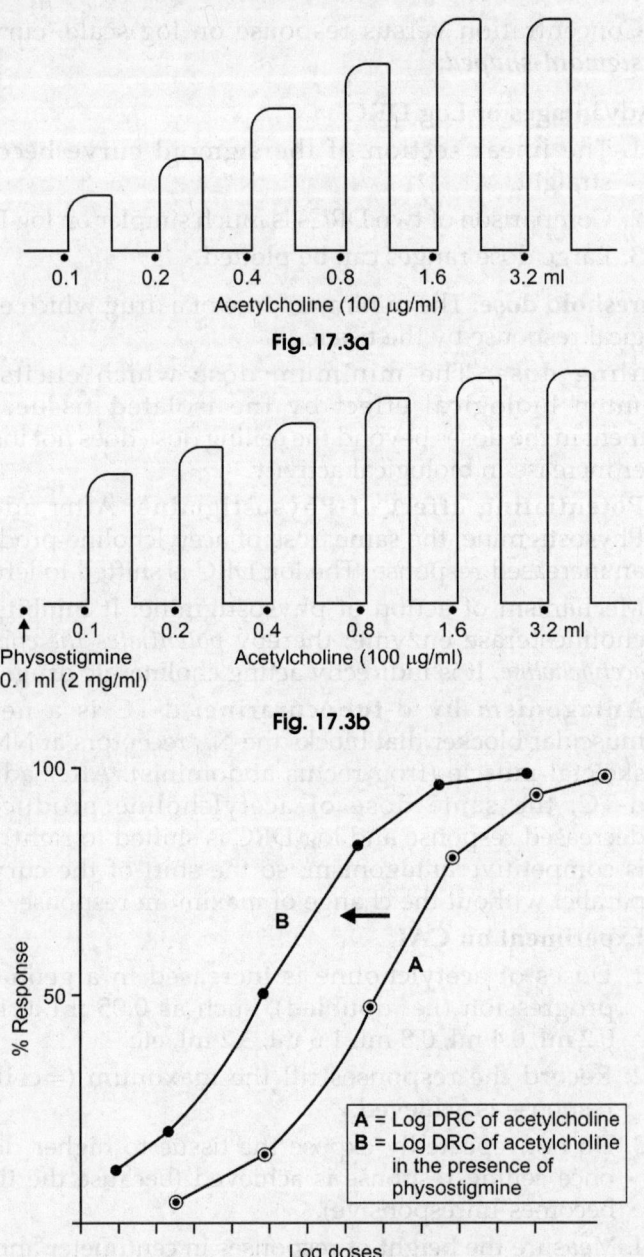

Fig. 17.3c: Potentiation effect of physostigmine (log DRC is shifted to left).

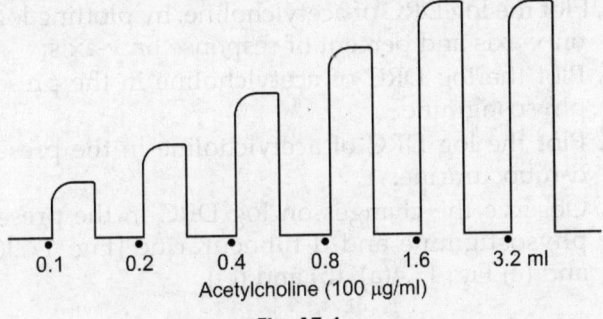

Fig. 17.4a

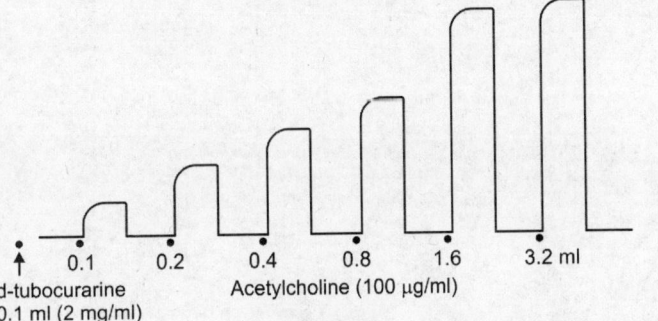

Fig. 17.4b

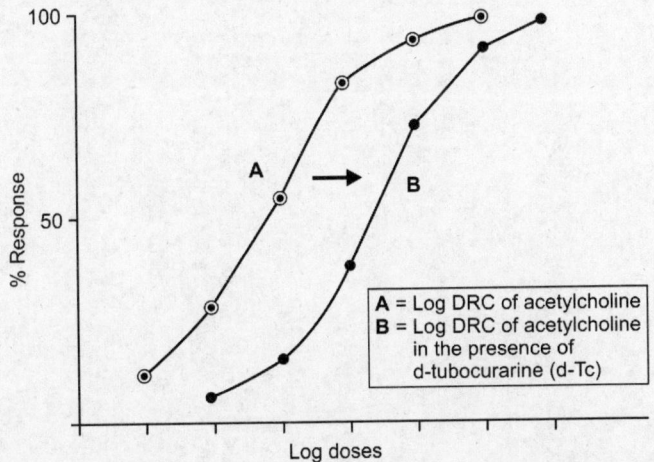

Fig. 17.4c: Antagonism effect of d-TC (Log DRC is shifted to right)

5. Plot the log DRC of acetylcholine, by plotting log doses on x-axis and percent of response on y-axis.

6. Plot the log DRC of acetylcholine in the presence of physostigmine.

7. Plot the log DRC of acetylcholine in the presence of d-tubocurarine.

8. Observe the changes on log DRC in the presence of physostigmine and d-tubocurarine [Fig. 17.3(a), (b) and (c) Fig. 17.4(a), (b) and (c)].

18

Effect of Cardiac Stimulants and Cardiac Depressants on Isolated and Perfused Frog's Heart

INTRODUCTION

The heart is innervated by both sympathetic and parasympathetic nervous system. Postganglionic sympathetic neurons supply the SA node and myocardial tissues of atria and ventricles. The postganglionic parasympathetic neurons supply the SA node, atria and A-V conduction tissue. Ventricular tissue have no parasympathetic innervations. Effect of drugs on the heart depends on the balance between sympathetic and parasympathetic activity and the drug administered. Activation of sympathetic system exerts positive chronotropic, positive inotropic and positive dromotropic action. The reverse is true with parasympathetic system.

Cardiac stimulants and depressants: They may act indirectly via adrenergic or cholinergic receptors or may act directly.

Cardiac stimulants: Sympathomimetics such as adrenaline, noradrenaline, dopamine, phenylephrine, methylxanthines and calcium salts.

Cardiac depressants: Cholinomimetics, beta blockers, calcium channel blockers, potassium and magnesium salts.

Physiology of Cardiac Muscle

- Exhibit contractility, excitability, conductivity and autorhythmicity.

133

- Autorhythmicity is due to presence of specialized pacemaker tissue: SA node, AV node, A-V bundle and Purkinje fibres.
- Cardiac receptors are β_1 adrenergic and M2 muscarinic.
- **Effect of sympathomimetics/adrenaline:** Agonists of β_1 adrenergic receptors (GPCR) exerts
  - i. **Positive chronotropic effect (increased HR):** By increasing the slope of slow diastolic depolarization in cells of SA node.
  - ii. **Positive inotropic effect (increased force of contraction):** $\hat{a}_1$ adrenergic receptors (GPCR) act through Gs protein, activate adenylate cyclase, increase cyclic AMP which phosphorylates protein kinases and troponin and activate calcium channels promoting calcium influx that results in increased force of contraction and cardiac output increases.
  - iii. **Positive dromotropic effect (increased conduction velocity):** Through AV node A-V bundle and increased refractory period.
  - iv. **Tachyarrhythmias may occur.**
- **Effect of cholinomimetics/acetylcholine/vagal stimulation:** Muscarinic M2 receptor agonists exert
  - i. **Negative chronotropic effect (decreased HR):** M2 receptor is a GPCR, acts through Gi protein, opens K^+ channels, inhibits adenylate cyclase and decreases cyclic AMP, resulting in hyperpolarization of SA nodal cells and decreased rate of diastolic depolarization, and reduced HR.
  - ii. **Negative inotropic effect (decreased force of contraction):** Due to reduced cyclic AMP and reduced Ca^{++} influx in myocardial cells.
  - iii. **Negative dromotropic effect (decreased conduction velocity):** At A-V node and Purkinje fibres and increased refractory period.
  - iv. **Bradyarrhythmias may occur**
- **Effect of calcium and potassium:**
  - i. Increase in calcium in ECF increases myocardial contractility and heart may stop in systole (=systolic arrest).

   ii. Decrease in calcium has opposite effect.

   iii. Increase in potassium in ECF (= hyperkalemia) leads to decrease in RMP, loss of conductivity, contractility and excitability and heart may stop in diastole (= diastolic arrest).

Objective: To study the effects of cardiac stimulants and cardiac depressants on isolated perfused frog heart.

Requirements: Animal: Frog

Physiological salt solution: Frog Ringer solution.

Equipment: Pithing needle, dissection instruments, Syme's cannula, Starling's heart lever, perfusion bottle, recording apparatus, pin-hook and thread.

Drugs

Adrenaline	10 µg/ml (0.1, 0.2 ml)
Calcium chloride	10 mg/ml (0.2 ml)
Propranolol	50 µg/ml (0.1, 0.2 ml)
Acetylcholine	10 µg/ml (0.1, 0.2 ml)
Potassium chloride	10 mg/ml (0.2 ml)
Atropine sulphate	50 µg/ml (0.1, 0.2 ml)

Procedure: Steps
1. Pith the medium-sized frog (double pithing)
2. Frog is pinned on the board in a tray.
3. Abdominal wall is removed by a V-shaped incision from pelvis to pectoral girdle.
4. Heart is exposed and pericardium removed by fine scissors.
5. Hook the ventricle at its apex and attach with a thread on Starling's heart lever.
6. Place a thread under exposed inferior vena cava and cut a slit in the direction of heart.

7. Insert Syme's cannula (filled with frog Ringer solution) through the slit and tie it firmly.
8. Start perfusion of frog Ringer solution.
9. The heart will bulge due to perfusion.
10. Cut the two truncus arteriosus so that fluid comes out.
11. The perfusion rate is maintained at 40 drops/min.
12. Contractions are recorded by Starling's heart lever on the drum.
13. The drugs are injected into the rubber tubing nearest to the cannula.
14. Control/normal tracing should be recorded before adding next drug.
15. Observe the effect of cardiac stimulants and depressants.

Experiment on CAL

Steps

1. Control tracing
2. Adrenaline (10 mcg/ml, 0.2 ml)
3. Control tracing
4. CaCl$_2$ (10 mg/ml, 0.2 ml)
5. Control tracing
6. Acetylcholine (10 mcg/ml, 0.2 ml)
7. Control tracing
8. KCl (10 mg/ml, 0.2 ml)
9. Control tracing
10. Propranolol (50 mcg/ml, 0.2 ml) plus adrenaline (10 mcg/ml, 0.2 ml)
11. Control tracing
12. Propranolol (50 mcg/ml, 0.2 ml) plus CaCl$_2$ (10 mg/ml, 0.2 ml)
13. Control tracing
14. Atropine (50 mcg/ml, 0.2 ml) plus acetylcholine (10 mcg/ml, 0.2 ml)
15. Control tracing
16. Atropine (50 mcg/ml, 0.2 ml) plus KCl (10 mg/ml, 0.2 ml)

Observation Table

S.N.	Drug	HR (bpm)	Tone ↑ or ↓ or unchanged	Amplitude ↑ or ↓ or unchanged

Basal HR =.........(bpm)

Point to remember: Receptor antagonists (blockers), do not produce any effect in this experiment, because there is no resting tone either sympathetic or parasympathetic, since both have been completely destroyed by pithing. If blockers produce any response, the possibility of incomplete pithing must be considered.

Discussion

Three parameters are recorded.
1. **Tone of muscle:** Partial contraction of muscle on tracing, indicated by baseline of tracing. Thus, increased tone is shown by rise of baseline and decreased tone by fall of baseline. *(inotropic effect).*
2. **Amplitude:** Force of contraction. Total height of curve indicates amplitude *(inotropic effect).*
3. **Heart rate:** Number of contractions per minute *(chronotropic effect).*

Note: *Systolic and diastolic arrest may occur on large doses of* $CaCl_2$ *and on large doses of KCl respectively.*

Inferences

On the basis of effect, drugs can be divided into two categories.
1. **Stimulant:**   Direct acting—$CaCl_2$
   Indirect acting—adrenaline
2. **Depressant:**   Direct acting—KCl
   Indirect acting—acetylcholine

Precautions

1. Thread should be vertical and lever should be horizontal
2. Ratio between long and short arm of lever should be 10:1.

Composition of frog's Ringer solution	
Sodium chloride	6.5 g
Potassium chloride	0.14 g
Calcium chloride	0.12 g
Sodium dihydrogen phosphate	0.008 g
Sodium bicarbonate	0.2 g
Glucose	2.0 g
Distilled water	up to 1000 ml

Graph 18.1: Cardiac stimulant action of adrenaline

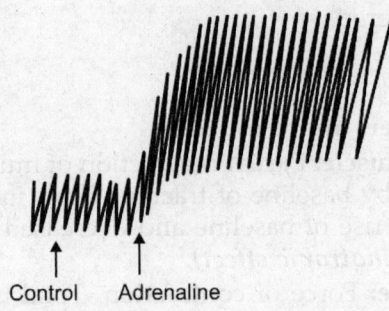

Control   Adrenaline

Graph 18.2: Cardiac stimulant action of $CaCl_2$

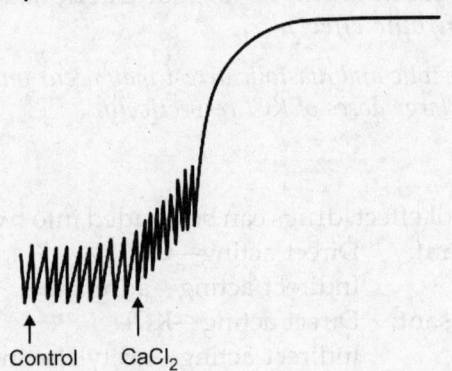

Control $CaCl_2$

Discussion about the drugs

SN	Drug	HR	Tone	Amplitude	Rhythm	Comment
1.	Adrenaline	↑	↑	↑	Regular/heart may stop in systole (high dose)	Cardiac stimulant, act on β receptors
2.	CaCl$_2$	↑/0	↑↑↑	↑/0	Heart stops in systole	Direct acting stimulant
3.	Acetylcholine	↓	↓	↓	Regular/heart may stop in diastole (at high dose)	Cardiac depressant, act on M2 receptors
4.	KCl	↓	↓↓↓	↓	Heart stops in diastole	Direct acting depressant
5.	Propranolol + Adrenaline	No change	No change	No change	Regular	Propranolol is a β-blocker, so adrenaline is unable to show its stimulant action
6.	Propranolol + CaCl$_2$	↑/0	↑↑↑	↑/0	Heart stops in systole	Effect of CaCl$_2$ is not blocked by propranolol
7.	Atropine + acetylcholine	No change	No change	No change	Regular	Atropine is muscarinic antagonist, so acetylcholine is unable to show its depressant action
8.	Atropine + KCl	↓/0	↓↓↓	↓/0	Heart stops in diastole	Effect of KCl is not blocked by atropine

Graph 18.3: Cardiac depressant action of acetylcholine

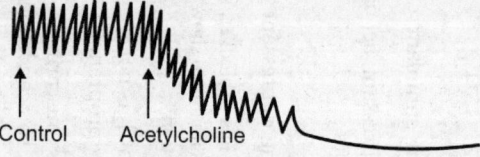

Graph 18.4: Cardiac depressant action of KCl

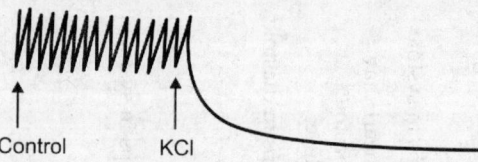

Graph 18.5: Blockade of cardiac stimulant action of adrenaline in the presence of propranolol

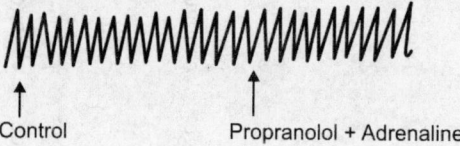

Graph 18.6: Cardiac stimulant action of CaCl$_2$ even in the presence of propranolol

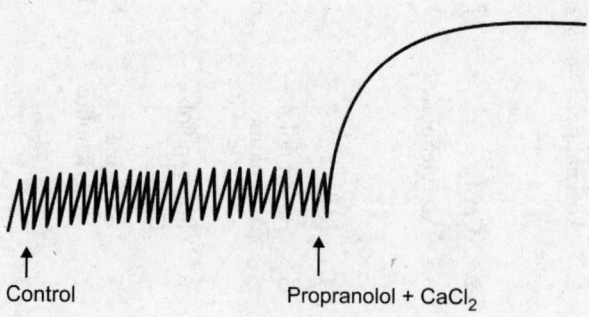

Graph 18.7: Blockade of cardiac depressant action of acetylcholine in the presence of atropine

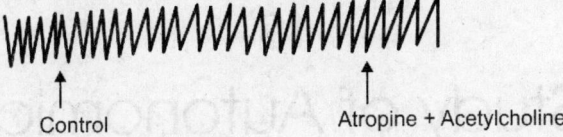

Control   Atropine + Acetylcholine

Graph 18.8: Cardiac depressant action of KCl, even in the presence of atropine

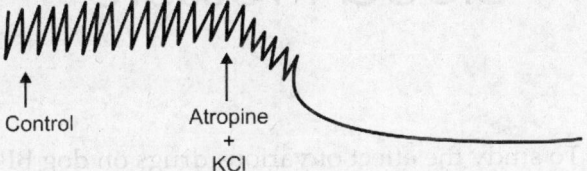

Control   Atropine
                              +
                            KCl

19

Study of Autonomic Drugs on Mammalian Blood Pressure

Object: To study the effect of various drugs on dog BP.
1. Effects of epinephrine, norepinephrine and isoprenaline on BP
2. Dale's vasomotor reversal and re-reversal
3. Tachyphylaxis
4. Nicotinic/ganglionic action of acetylcholine

Animal: Dog/Cat

Apparatus: Research kymograph/computer and data acquisition system, operation table, U-shaped mercury manometer, tuberculin syringe, burette, arterial, venous and tracheal cannula, connecting rubber tube, dissecting instruments, cotton and thread.

Drugs Required

Epinephrine = 2 microgram/kg, 1–3 microgram/kg
Norepinephrine = 3 microgram/kg, 2–5 microgram/kg
Isoprenaline = 3 microgram/kg, 2–5 microgram/kg
Acetylcholine = 5 microgram/kg, 2–10 microgram/kg
Atropine = 1000 microgram/kg, 500–1000 microgram/kg

For observing nicotinic action of acetylcholine, first we fully antagonize muscarinic receptors by giving a large dose of atropine (2000 microgram/kg) followed by 5–10 times higher dose of acetylcholine (50 microgram/kg).

Phentolamine=1000 microgram/kg

Propranolol=1000 microgram/kg

Ephedrine= 100 microgram/kg, 100–200 microgram/kg

Saline (0.9%)

Chloralose (anaesthetic agent)= 80–100 mg/kg body weght.

Procedure: A healthy dog is weighed and anaesthetized with pentobarbitone sodium (25 mg/kg IV) or chloralose (100 mg/kg IV). After the animal has been anaesthetized, it is mounted on operation table in supine position. Four limbs are tied to four corners of operation table. After that femoral vein is exposed in thigh region and venous cannula is inserted in the vein. Venous cannula is connected to a burette with the help of rubber tubing which contains normal saline. This route is used for injecting drugs IV.

After that a midline incision is given in neck. Skin and fascia reflected, muscles are separated and trachea is exposed. After exposing trachea, search for carotid artery lying in deeper tissue on the side of trachea. An arterial cannula (heparinised) is inserted in the carotid artery and this cannula is connected to a mercury manometer with the help of pressure rubber tubing. This set is used for recording of BP on drum. A partial transverse cut is given in trachea and a Y-shaped tracheal cannula is inserted in the lumen of trachea and connected to a respiratory pump.

The drugs are given IV through femoral vein.

Experiment on CAL

- **Experiment (1): Steps:** Epinephrine → phentolamine → epinephrine → propranolol → epinephrine
- **Experiment (2): Steps:** Norepinephrine → phentolamine → norepinephrine → propranolol → norepinephrine
- **Experiment (3): Steps:** Isoprenaline → phentolamine → isoprenaline → propranolol → isoprenaline
- **Experiment (4): Steps:** Ephedrine → ephedrine → ephedrine → ephedrine → ephedrine
- **Experiment (5): Steps:** Acetylcholine (5 mcg/kg) → atropine (2000 mcg/kg) → acetylcholine (50 mcg/kg)

Observation Table 1

SN	Drug	HR (bpm)	Mean BP (mmHg)	Remarks
1.	Epinephrine			
2.	Phentolamine			
3.	Epinephrine			
4.	Propranolol			
5.	Epinephrine			

Basal HR=   Basal mean BP=

Observation Table 2

SN	Drug	HR (bpm)	Mean BP (mmHg)	Remarks
1.	Norepinephrine			
2.	Phentolamine			
3.	Norepinephrine			
4.	Propranolol			
5.	Norepinephrine			

Basal HR=   Basal mean BP=

Observation Table 3

SN	Drug	HR (bpm)	Mean BP (mmHg)	Remarks
1.	Isoprenaline			
2.	Phentolamine			
3.	Isoprenaline			
4.	Propranolol			
5.	Isoprenaline			

Basal HR=   Basal mean BP=

Observation Table 4

SN	Drug	HR (bpm)	Mean BP (mmHg)	Remarks
1.	Ephedrine			
2.	Ephedrine			
3.	Ephedrine			
4.	Ephedrine			
5.	Ephedrine			

Basal HR=   Basal mean BP=

Observation Table 5

SN	Drug	HR (bpm)	Mean BP (mmHg)	Remarks
1.	Acetylcholine (5 mcg/kg)			
2.	Atropine (2000 mcg/kg)			
3.	Acetylcholine (50 mcg/kg)			

Basal HR=   Basal mean BP=

Graph: Experiment 19.1

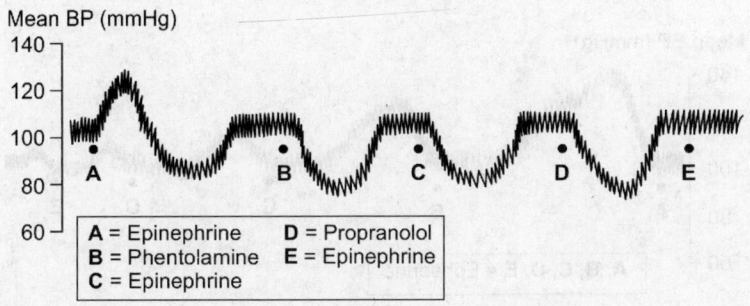

Mean BP (mmHg)

A = Epinephrine   D = Propranolol
B = Phentolamine   E = Epinephrine
C = Epinephrine

Graph: Experiment 19.2

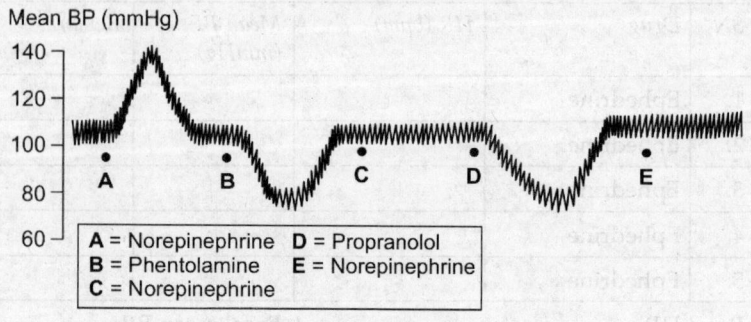

Mean BP (mmHg)

A = Norepinephrine   D = Propranolol
B = Phentolamine   E = Norepinephrine
C = Norepinephrine

Graph: Experiment 19.3

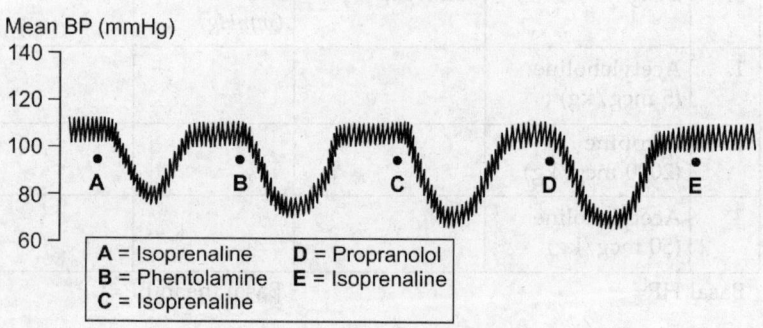

Mean BP (mmHg)

A = Isoprenaline   D = Propranolol
B = Phentolamine   E = Isoprenaline
C = Isoprenaline

Graph: Experiment 19.4

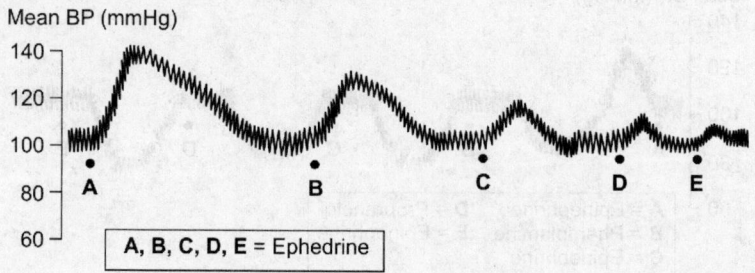

Mean BP (mmHg)

A, B, C, D, E = Ephedrine

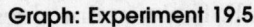

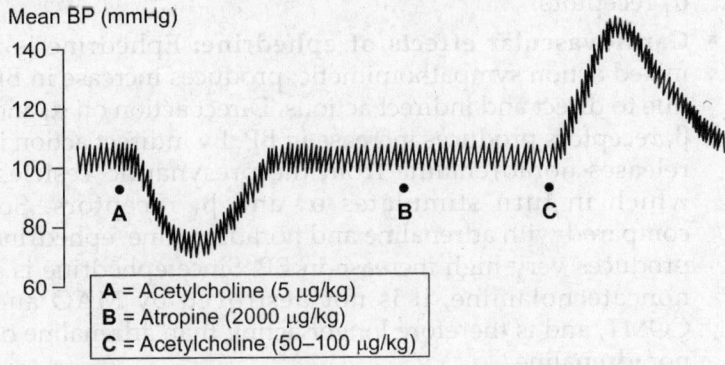

Graph: Experiment 19.5

Mean BP (mmHg)

A = Acetylcholine (5 µg/kg)
B = Atropine (2000 µg/kg)
C = Acetylcholine (50–100 µg/kg)

Discussion

- **Cardiovascular effects of epinephrine or adrenaline:** Adrenaline produces biphasic response in blood pressure. The initial increase in blood pressure is due to the action of epinephrine on α_1 and β_1 receptors (and tachycardia due to β_1 action), action on β_2 receptors produces vasodilatation of blood vessels of skeletal muscles resulting in slight fall in BP. (At large concentration α_1 action predominates while at low concentration β_2 action predominates).

- **Cardiovascular effects of norepinephrine or noradrenaline:** Noradrenaline acts on α_1 receptors producing vasoconstriction and peripheral vascular resistance increases. It acts on β_1 receptors producing increase in cardiac contraction and rate, thereby increasing the cardiac output. Thus BP increases (BP= cardiac output X peripheral resistance). Noradrenaline does not have action on β_2 receptors, thereby no fall in BP. Ultimate effect of noradrenaline on heart rate is initial tachycardia followed by bradycardia (reflex bradycardia caused by noradrenaline is due to vagus nerve effect as a result of rise of mean BP).

- **Cardiovascular effects of isoprenaline:** Isoprenaline acts on β_1 receptors and produces tachycardia. But its action on β_2 receptors produce vasodilatation resulting in lowering of peripheral resistance which is responsible for fall in diastolic BP. Isoprenaline does not have action on α_1 receptors.

- **Cardiovascular effects of ephedrine:** Ephedrine is a mixed action sympathomimetic, produces increase in BP due to direct and indirect actions. Direct action on α_1 and β_1 receptors produces increase in BP. By indirect action it releases noradrenaline from the presynaptic vesicles, which in turn stimulates α_1 and β_1 receptors. So, compared with adrenaline and noradrenaline, ephedrine produces very high increase in BP. Since ephedrine is a noncatecholamine, it is not destroyed by MAO and COMT, and is therefore longer acting than adrenaline or noradrenaline.

- **Cardiovascular effects of phentolamine:** Phentolamine is reversible non-selective α blocker. Due to blockade of vasoconstrictor α receptor it leads to vasodilatation and fall in PVR and BP. Reflex tachycardia occurs due to fall in mean BP and increased release of noradrenaline due to blockade of presynaptic α_2 receptors.

- **Cardiovascular effects of propranolol:** It is a non-selective beta blocker blocks both β_1 and β_2 receptors, decreases heart rate, force of contraction (at higher doses) and cardiac output. Propranolol causes fall in BP due to negative chronotropic, negative inotropic action and reduced cardiac output.

- **Dale's vasomotor reversal and re-reversal:** Rapid IV injection of adrenaline acts on $\alpha1$ receptors, produces rise of systolic, diastolic and mean BP initially. After some time when concentration of adrenaline is reduced, adrenaline acts on β_2 receptors, produces vasodilatation, reduces mean and diastolic BP. This is called as biphasic response of adrenaline. If α receptor are blocked, by α blocker, then adrenaline elicits only fall in diastolic BP. This is called vasomotor reversal of Dale. Norepinephrine does not exhibit Dale's vasomotor reversal phenomenon because it has a predominant α action with negligible β_2 action. Further administration of beta blocker (propranolol) will cause re-reversal of vasomotor reversal effect.

- **Cardiovascular effects of acetylcholine:** Acetylcholine acts on M3 receptors in blood vessels and produces vasodilatation and decrease in peripheral resistance and subsequent fall in BP. M3 receptors are present on vascular endothelial cells. Vasodilatation is primarily mediated through the release of endothelium derived relaxing factor (EDRF) or nitric oxide (NO). Acetylcholine also acts on M2 receptors in heart and decreases the heart rate and force of contraction. Bradycardia is due to the direct action on M2 receptors on SA nodes of heart due to reduced rate of diastolic depolarization.

- **Cardiovascular effects of atropine:** Initial bradycardia followed by tachycardia. No consistent effect on BP.

- **Nicotinic/ganglionic action of acetylcholine:** Acetylcholine has both muscarinic and nicotinic actions . Due to muscarinic agonistic action it reduces heart rate (M2) and BP (M2, M3). Prior atropinization followed by a heavy dose of acetylcholine results in nicotinic or ganglionic action of acetylcholine in BP experiment. In this effect BP increases, since muscarinic receptor are blocked by atropine, only nicotinic action of acetylcholine is seen due to stimulation of N_N receptors of autonomic ganglia and release of catecholamines from adrenal medulla and sympathetic ganglia.

- **Tachyphylaxis:** Reduction in response to a drug when it is repeatedly given at short intervals. It is also called acute tolerance. It is due to exhaustion of the noradrenaline available for displacement from the neuronal pool. Seen with ephedrine and tyramine.

Bibliography

1. Bhavana Srivastava: Experimental Pharmacology, 1st edition, New Central Book Agency (P) Ltd., Kolkata, 2007.
2. Brunton LL, Chabner BA and Knollman BC, Eds: Goodman and Gilman's The Pharmacological Basis of Therapeutics, 12th edition, McGraw-Hill, New York, USA, 2011.
3. Devi J Sujatha: Experimental Pharmacology for undergraduates and postgraduates, 1st edition, Jaypee Brothers Medical Publishers (P) Ltd., New Delhi, 2013.
4. Garg GR and Arya S: Experimental Pharmacology for undergraduates, 1st edition, CBS Publishers and Distributors Pvt. Ltd., New Delhi, 2005.
5. Ghosh MN: Fundamentals of Experimental Pharmacology, 6th edition, Hilton and Company, Kolkata, 2015.
6. Medhi Bikash and Prakash A: Practical manual of Experimental and Clinical Pharmacology, 1st edition, Jaypee Brothers Medical Publishers (P) Ltd., New Delhi, 2010.
7. Sharma HL and Sharma KK: Principles of Pharmacology, 2nd edition, Paras Medical Publishers, Hyderabad, 2011.
8. Tripathi KD: Essentials of Medical Pharmacology, 7th edition, Jaypee Brothers Medical Publishers (P) Ltd., New Delhi, 2013.

Index

153

Reader's Notes

Reader's Notes

Reader's Notes